Atlas of Occupational Health and Disease

Atlas of Occupational Health and Disease

Nerys R. Williams
*Consultant Occupational Physician and
Honorary Senior Clinical Lecturer,
Institute of Occupational Health,
Birmingham, UK*

John Harrison
*Clinical Director Occupational Health
Occupational Health Department
Hammersmith Hospitals NHS Trust
London, UK*

131149

ARNOLD

A Member of the Hodder Headline Group
LONDON

First published in Great Britain in 2004 by
Arnold, a member of the Hodder Headline Group,
338 Euston Road, London NW1 3BH

http://www.arnoldpublishers.com

Distributed in the United States of America by
Oxford University Press Inc.,
198 Madison Avenue, New York, NY10016
Oxford is a registered trademark of Oxford University Press

British Library Cataloguing in Publication Data
A catalogue record for this book is available from the British Library

Library of Congress Cataloging-in-Publication Data
A catalog record for this book is available from the Library of Congress

ISBN 0340740698

1 2 3 4 5 6 7 8 9 10

Commissioning Editor: Joanna Koster
Project Editor: Zelah Pengilley
Production Controller: Deborah Smith
Cover Design: Lee-May Lim

Typeset in 9 on 11pt Sabon by Phoenix Photosetting, Chatham, Kent
Printed and bound in Italy.

What do you think about this book? Or any other Arnold title? Please send your comments to

feedback.arnold@hodder.co.uk

Contents

Foreword

The effects of work on health has been a subject of interest since the social reformers of the 19th century campaigned against the worst vicissitudes of the Industrial Revolution. Clinicians showed a growing interest in the subject in the last century following the lead of Thomas Legge and Donald Hunter. In addition to the desire to improve workers' health and to prevent others from becoming ill, those interested and specializing in Occupational Health also have a fascination for viewing the worker at work. It is a time-consuming task but is there really any substitute for seeing the workplace in order to assess that worker's problem and those of their mates?

For the busy clinician in hospital or general practice, the luxury of a trip to the workplace is rare indeed. In an effort to provide some pictorial substitute to aid these health practitioners, Nerys Williams and John Harrison have assembled an astonishing array of photographs of workplaces and work-related diseases. The structure of the content follows the format of the ninth edition of *Hunter's Diseases of Occupations*, and the atlas can thus be used in conjunction with it or independently.

I believe that even our illustrious forebears Bernardino Ramazzini and Charles Turner Thackrah would have valued such an atlas on their bookshelves!

Professor Malcolm Harrington
July 2003

Preface

The practice of occupational medicine and the promotion of occupational health require an ability to make a clinical assessment of people (workers) and to assess their places of work. Ultimately, the aim is to ensure that workers can earn a living without jeopardizing their health. However, achieving good occupational health and what has been called 'work ability' is a multi-stage process involving many different stakeholders. They may be general medical practitioners, primary care nurses, hospital specialists, members of the occupational health team, engineers, managers or human resources officers. The list is not exhaustive. We should not forget the general public and their elected representatives, who make decisions about resource allocation as well as enacting new legislation. Work and the ability to work is something that affects all of us at some time in our lives. Unfortunately, awareness of workplace hazards and of the risks to health of working practices and environments is lacking amongst many of the stakeholders. This is despite the plethora of information that is available.

Our aim, in compiling this book, has been to present different aspects of occupational health in a visual format to try to bring this important subject to life. Occupational health is about people and about workplaces. We have tried to include as many pictures as possible to portray the panoply of working environments. Of course, we could never hope to achieve this completely, but it has been surprisingly difficult to find good photographs of workplaces or workers, or of occupational diseases. This has caused us some concern because the world of work is always changing and valuable occupational health records may be lost forever. It is our hope that this book will encourage contributions, in the future, either from the so-called developed world or from other parts of the world, where there may be good examples of working life in a global economy.

The *Atlas of Occupational Health and Disease* is intended to be an accessible and useful source of information. It is not a textbook as the contents have been limited by the availability of pictures and by the desire to limit accompanying texts to a maximum of about 150 words. The chapter headings are broadly the same as those in the ninth edition of *Hunter's Disease of Occupations* and readers wishing more detailed information about the entries are advised to consult this reference book. We hope that the atlas will prove to be useful for anyone studying for an occupational health qualification, or indeed, any qualification that is based on a syllabus that includes health, health promotion, the diagnosis and management of disease, rehabilitation or the recruitment and retention of workers.

Nerys Williams
John Harrison

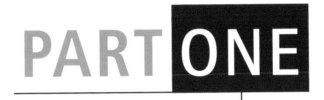

PART ONE

DISEASES ASSOCIATED WITH CHEMICAL AGENTS

(a) Beryllium

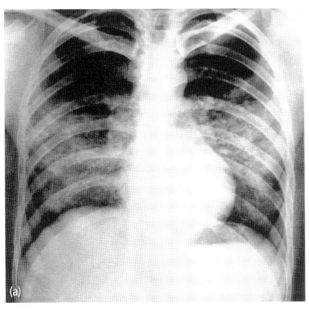 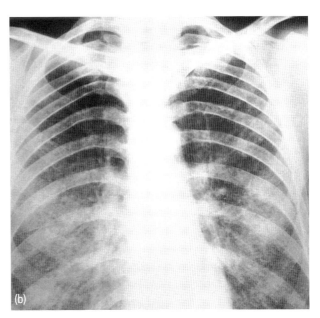

Figure 1.1 (a) Acute beryllium disease in a male metallurgist. Copyright the late Harriet Hardy. (b) Chronic beryllium disease in a fluorescent lamp worker showing widespread and large ill-defined opacities in the middle and lower zones. Copyright W. Jones Williams. Both (a) and (b) reproduced with permission from *Occupational Lung Disorders*, 3rd edition, edited by W. Raymond Parkes, published in 1994 by Butterworth-Heinemann Ltd.

Exposure to beryllium and beryllium-containing compounds occurs in metal and alloy workers, ceramic manufacturing, the electronics and space industries and in laboratory workers. Historically, it also occurred in fluorescent lamp workers, but this process ceased around 1950. Acute exposure to the metal produces non-respiratory symptoms such as conjunctivitis, corneal ulceration and allergic dermatitis. Respiratory disease usually follows excessive exposure and produces tracheitis and bronchitis with a chemical pneumonia. This latter condition can have a fulminant course but generally acute disease resolves completely, only rarely progressing to the chronic state. It is important to note that the x-ray findings lag behind clinical features by a few weeks. A diffuse haziness develops first, followed by widespread ill-defined opacities (see figure a). As the patient recovers, the opacities clear and in most cases the x-ray returns to normal within a few months.

Chronic beryllium disease differs markedly from the acute condition. It is an insidious illness, developing after up to 20 years of variable exposure. It primarily affects the lungs, but sensitization is often found as well. Usually the presenting feature is increasing breathlessness, which may be accompanied by an irritating cough. In advanced disease there is weight loss and anorexia. Lung function test findings are not specific, but pulmonary densities may be seen on x-ray and are usually bilateral (see figure b). The condition can result in severe disabling disease, particularly when exacerbations are accompanied by fever. In order to diagnose the condition, there must be a history of exposure and the presence of beryllium in tissues. Findings such as granulomas and hypersensitivity are not specific as the main condition to exclude is sarcoidosis. Lymphocyte transformation tests may be helpful in identifying sensitivity to the disease, as correlation with the condition is good.

(b) Cadmium

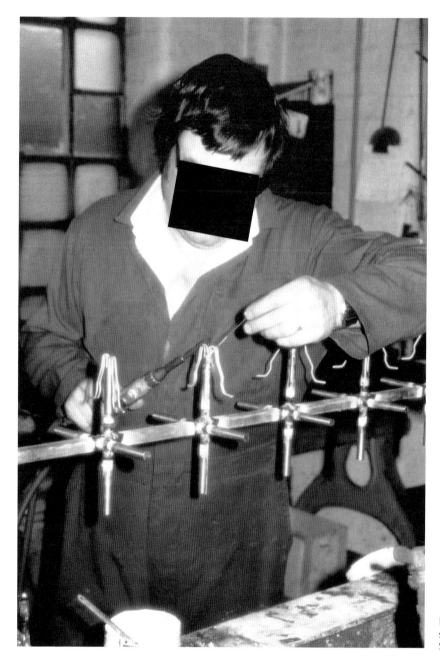

Figure 1.2 Jig maker using cadmium-containing silver solder. Copyright Health & Safety Laboratory, Sheffield, UK. Reproduced with permission.

Cadmium is a bluish white metal that is resistant to corrosion. It is used in the manufacture of bearing alloys and is added to silver as an ingredient in brazing alloys and in solders. Cadmium is also used in electroplating and in the formation of pigments for paints, rubber, plastics etc.

Acute poisoning may result from the inhalation of cadmium fumes, producing symptoms of headache, cough and shortness of breath. Renal necrosis has also been reported in severe poisoning. Less severe inhalation of cadmium oxide fumes results in metal fume fever, and chronic exposure is associated with yellow staining of the teeth, rhinitis and anosmia from atrophy of the nasal mucosa.

Chronic exposure also produces proteinuria (of tubular type), indicating renal damage and emphysema; both conditions may develop years after exposure has ceased but, given the half-life of cadmium (10 years), individuals usually continue to have high levels of cadmium in their urine, indicating high levels of exposure previously.

(c) Chromium

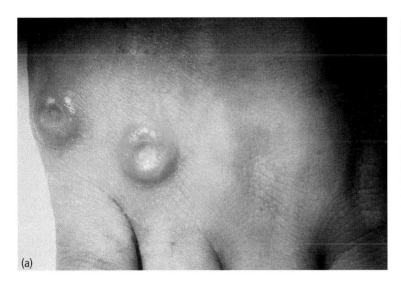 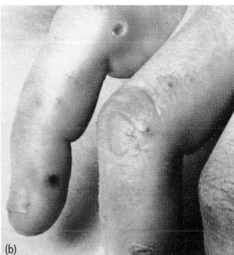

Figure 1.3 (a) and (b) Chromium toxicity: chrome ulcers on the hand and fingers. Courtesy of the Health & Safety Executive, UK. Crown copyright material is reproduced with the permission of the Controller of Her Majesty's Stationery Office.

Chromium compounds are used widely in industry, e.g. for dyeing in the textile industry, for tanning and as pigments. In addition to causing contact dermatitis, chrome ulcers (or 'chrome holes') may occur in the skin. These ulcers have a punched-out appearance and may be painful, particularly if they become secondarily infected. The ulcers usually take 2–3 weeks to heal, leaving a permanent scar. Similar lesions occur due to contact with mercury fulminate. Exposure to hexavalent chromium may also cause occupational asthma and an increased risk of lung cancer.

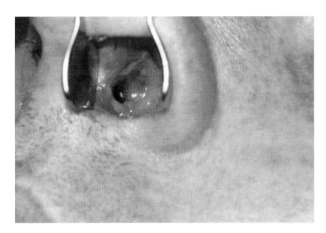

Figure 1.4 Perforation of the nasal septum due to chromium (VI). Courtesy of the Health & Safety Executive, UK. Crown copyright material is reproduced with the permission of the Controller of Her Majesty's Stationery Office.

The commonest occupational cause of nasal perforation is associated with exposure to hexavalent chromium compounds. Perforation, which is preceded by ulceration, is a recognized hazard for chrome platers and it is in this group that case reports dating back to 1902 can be found. The interval between first exposure to the development of ulceration and perforation has been reported to be between 6 and 12 months, although nasal ulcers have been reported after only a few days of plating activity. Initially, workers may complain of pain and some nasal bleeding. However, once the ulcer has progressed to perforation, bleeding and pain cease. The resulting hole in the septum may be asymptomatic or may lead to a whistling noise on breathing. If the worker is removed from exposure at the ulcer stage, healing occurs, leaving permanent scarring, usually in Little's area. Perforations do not repair themselves spontaneously, although surgical closure may be undertaken if a worker leaves the industry.

Perforation of the nasal septum can also occur as a consequence of occupational exposure to mercury fulminate, arsenic, ruthenium and platinum salts. It has been reported following nasal steroid therapy, and may result from local trauma, cocaine inhalation, postoperatively (such as after a sub-mucous resection) and in association with granulomatous diseases such as Wegener's granulomatosis.

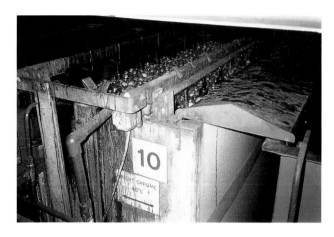

Figure 1.5 Plating tank containing chromium solution and cruffles. Copyright Mike Morgan, Health & Safety Executive, UK. Reproduced with permission.

The illustration shows a typical plating tank containing a chromium solution. If an electric current is passed through the solution, hydrogen gas is formed on the electrode; the gas bubbles rise and burst, releasing chrome mist into the air. The prevention of inhalation of the mist depends on the use of local exhaust ventilation and/or the use of a blanket of foam known as a mist suppressant. Cruffles, which resemble table tennis balls, are inadequate on their own. There is a legal requirement in the UK to measure levels of mist above tanks every 14 days by a prescribed method and also to check the adequacy of local exhaust ventilation.

(d) Cobalt

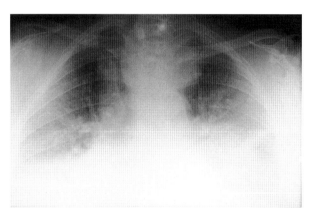

Figure 1.6 Chest x-ray showing enlarged thyroid and heart failure. Copyright John Harrison. Reproduced with permission.

Enlargement of the thyroid occurs relatively frequently, especially in women. Non-toxic goitres may be simple goitres due to iodine deficiency, or may occur due to goitrogens or may result from inborn errors of thyroid hormone synthesis. Cobalt is a goitrogen that occurs in the workplace. This silvery grey magnetic metal is used mainly in the manufacture of high-temperature alloys for jet engines. If ingested, between 5 and 45 per cent may be absorbed from the gut; if inhaled, about 30 per cent is absorbed from the respiratory tract. Cobalt inhibits tyrosine iodinase, thus preventing the synthesis of thyroxine. A large retrosternal goitre can deviate and compress the trachea. Hypothyroidism leads to the development of myxoedema, with characteristic features. The cardiovascular system is often affected and there may be a bradycardia and a low-voltage electrocardiogram (ECG). If untreated, heart failure may develop. Inhalation of cobalt may also give rise to an asthma-like condition called hard metal disease or an interstitial pulmonary fibrosis.

(e) Lead

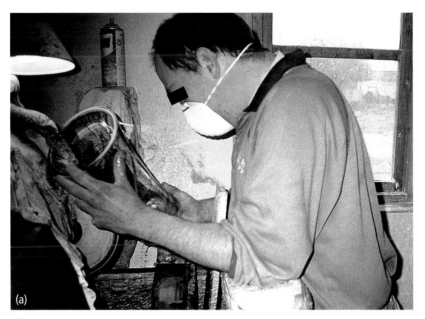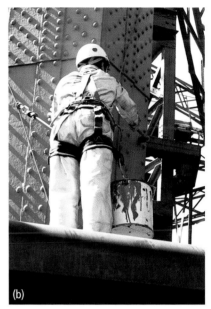

Figure 1.7 (a) Lead exposure during decorative glass cutting. (b) Use of lead paint in structural maintenance – The Eiffel Tower, Paris. Copyright Nerys R. Williams. Reproduced with permission.

Lead is still used in many industries: battery manufacture, as a pigment in paint and in the production of munitions. Exposure may occur occupationally and recreationally, e.g. in shooting ranges, and may be to lead fume (which is generally controlled by exhaust ventilation) or to lead dust. In the crystal glass industry, lead-containing glass is cut with a decorative pattern by an abrasive wheel, thus generating lead dust. The dust collects in water and is recycled, resulting in a rise in lead concentration. Workers may absorb the lead through inhalation when doing close work in conditions of inadequate extraction.

In addition to acute lead poisoning, which may cause symptoms such as colicky abdominal pain, constipation or diarrhoea and irritability, chronic poisoning may result in nephropathy, neuropathy and anaemia.

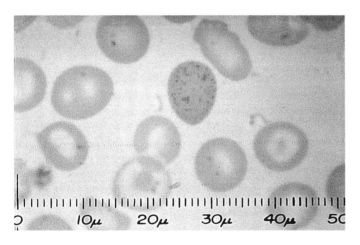

Figure 1.8 Red blood cells showing basophilic stippling. Copyright Anthony Yardley-Jones. Reproduced with permission.

There are few clinical signs that point to an unequivocal diagnosis of lead poisoning. The finding of an elevated level of lead in the blood, in isolation, is not synonymous with lead poisoning: the diagnosis is made based on the blood lead level and assessment of symptoms. Various haematological changes may be found in cases of lead poisoning, such as an elevated zinc protoporphyrin or anaemia (microcytic or normochromic). The appearance of basophilic stippling in red blood cells is a sign often recognized by haematologists as suggesting lead poisoning. However, it should be borne in mind that the appearance of stippling is not specific to the effects of lead; it may occur in severe anaemia, malignancy or malaria. The stippling is probably a combination of non-haem iron and other cell fragments, such as ferrigenous micelles, damaged mitochondria and RNA. It usually occurs at levels of blood lead in excess of 80 µg/100 mL, but it is not always found and there is a poor correlation with blood lead levels. The overall improvement in occupational hygiene has meant that basophilic stippling is now a rare finding on routine screening in Western Europe.

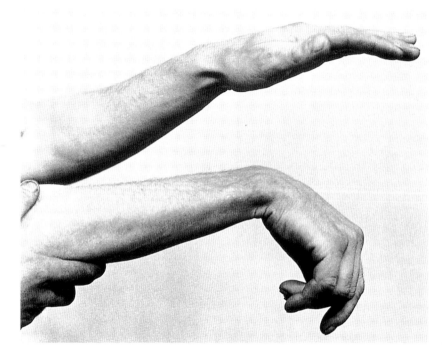

Figure 1.9 Wrist drop. Copyright Ian McCallum. Reproduced with permission.

Wrist drop may result from the development of a motor neuropathy or a radial nerve palsy. Lead poisoning is a well-described cause of motor peripheral neuropathy, in addition to the haematological changes that occur. Muscle weakness tends to occur in the muscles used most frequently and would be expected to be preceded by symptoms associated with poisoning, such as abdominal pain, colic and constipation. Improved protection from exposure to lead in developed countries, as a result of better occupational hygiene and health and safety legislation, means that lead neuropathy is now a very rare event.

(f) Mercury

Mercury is used industrially in the production of fungicides, biocides and special anti-fouling paints, in switch gear and laboratory and scientific apparatus including sphygmomanometers. It exists in many forms but all types cross biological membranes with ease and may be taken into the body by inhalation, ingestion or through the skin. Once in the body, inorganic mercury is absorbed into the bloodstream, where it is found equally distributed between the red cells and plasma (alkyl mercurial compounds differ in that they are concentrated in red cells). The main target organs are the kidneys and the central nervous system (CNS). Mercury is excreted in the urine and faeces, with a half-life of about 70 days in the body. Acute poisoning may produce symptoms related to the corrosive nature of many mercurial materials – pain and inflammation of the gastrointestinal or respiratory systems and signs of renal failure. Chronic exposure and poisoning produce classical symptoms of gingivitis, tremor and erethism. There may also be renal and CNS damage. Hypersalivation is also a feature, and the individual may complain of an unpleasant bitter taste in the mouth. The tremor is usually present at rest and can lead to difficulty writing. It may fluctuate in severity and be accompanied by ataxia. There is often an intentional cerebellar component to the CNS involvement and this makes the fine controlled action of handwriting difficult. Organic mercury poisoning may also present as a predominantly sensory peripheral neuropathy. Treatment involves chelation – by dimercaprol for inorganic mercury. Supervision of workers as well as the provision of instruction and training are essential to prevent occupational mercury poisoning; the regular analysis of urinary concentrations forms one component of an effective health surveillance programme for mercury-exposed workers.

(g) Selenium

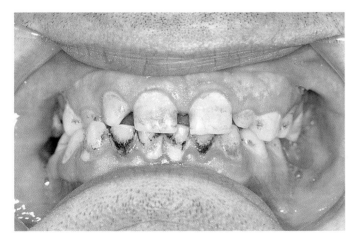

Figure 1.10 Poor dentition and gum health. Copyright John Harrison. Reproduced with permission.

Poor dentition may be due to a number of causes. It has been suggested that the ingestion of selenium leads to a higher rate of dental caries than is found generally. Evidence for this conclusion comes from a study comparing the dentition of children in two counties of Oregon, USA: Clatsop and Klamath. Children from Clatsop had poor dentition and more selenium in their urine than the children from Klamath, who had good dentition. Workers who have been exposed to selenium, e.g. in copper refineries, complain of a metallic taste in their mouth and the smell of garlic on their breath and in their sweat. There may be irritation of the nose and throat. It is advised that workers who have been exposed to selenium should be given ascorbic acid to remove the garlic odour.

(h) Silver

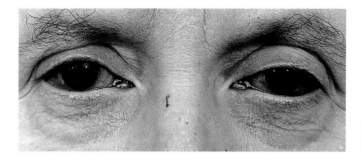

Figure 1.11 Argyrosis: silver deposition in the eyes. Courtesy of the Health & Safety Executive, UK. Crown copyright material is reproduced with the permission of the Controller of Her Majesty's Stationery Office.

Silver deposition in the eyes is known as argyrosis – a permanent grey discoloration that does not respond to chelating agents. There is no effect on visual acuity or on colour perception; however, the condition may be accompanied by the deposition of silver in the skin, either locally (as in the case of silversmiths) or generally – a condition known as argyria. Exposure to silver may take place in the photographic industry, in mirror manufacture and in the jewellery sector.

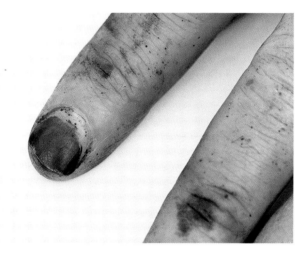

Figure 1.12 Silver nitrate staining of the fingernails. Courtesy of the Health & Safety Executive, UK. Crown copyright material is reproduced with the permission of the Controller of Her Majesty's Stationery Office.

Splash and spillage contact of silver compounds with the skin and nails also results in permanent external staining. The skin adopts a grey appearance over the area of contact that may darken in sunlight. Contact of the nails with soluble silver compounds such as silver nitrate produces the appearance shown here – permanent black staining and a sharp demarcation with normal-coloured nail as growth occurs. The condition is seen in individuals working in the photographic and refining industries and in plating.

Chapter 2 Gases

(a) Carbon monoxide

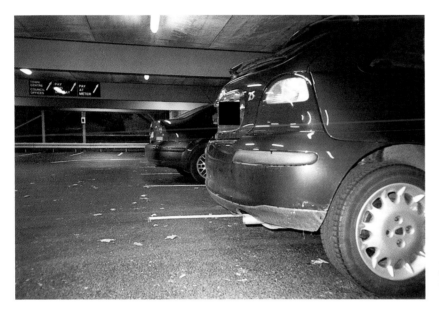

Figure 2.1 Carbon monoxide-containing car exhaust fumes in an underground car park – a risk for car park attendants. Copyright Nerys R. Williams. Reproduced with permission.

Carbon monoxide is a colourless, odourless and non-irritating gas which acts as an asphyxiant. Workers may be exposed in foundries, steel works and underground car parks, where attendants are particularly at risk. Domestically, poorly maintained boilers and gas appliances also account for many deaths from poisoning each year. Carbon monoxide is an asphyxiant because it combines with haemoglobin with an affinity 250 times greater than that of oxygen, thus causing the oxygen dissociation curve to shift to the left, making it more difficult for haemoglobin to give up oxygen to the tissues. Normal metabolism produces some carbon monoxide, but levels usually remain below 1 per cent. Cigarette smokers may have carboxyhaemoglobin (CHb) levels of up to 5–6 per cent, but in heavy smokers levels may rise as high as 10 per cent. Higher exposure may produce symptoms such as vomiting, headaches, weakness, tiredness, chest pain and palpitations, with individuals with anaemia and pre-existing heart disease particularly at risk. Often the condition is mistaken for a viral illness, but where more than one member of a household or an individual and their pet are affected, carbon monoxide poisoning should be suspected. Without effective treatment, long-term neuropsychiatric symptoms may result, so aggressive early treatment – oxygen supportive therapy and hyperbaric treatment – is indicated. Carbon monoxide can produce rapid unconsciousness; fatal levels are usually in excess of 50 per cent CHb in blood. The much-described classic cherry-red colour of the skin is rarely found, but if present suggests a CHb level in excess of 30 per cent. In pregnant women, studies have shown that fetal oxygenation changes with maternal levels as low as 5 per cent CHb; severe acute exposures can cause fetal death – hence pregnant women are advised to avoid occupational exposure to carbon monoxide.

See also 'Exposures during fires' (page 15).

(b) Ozone

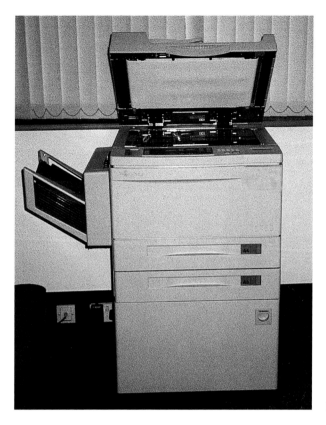

Figure 2.2 Photocopier. Copyright Nerys R. Williams. Reproduced with permission.

Photocopiers are now present in virtually every office. Health hazards related to their use are rare, but staff may complain of the machine emitting a fresh smell, which is irritating to the eyes and nose. This effect may be caused by ozone, which has an odour threshold well below any level likely to cause harm. The ozone is emitted when the filters in the machine need to be replaced. One report of lung disease related to exposure to used toner dust has not been further substantiated. All office equipment emits heat and can cause localized drying of the air, resulting in local low humidity and the development of low-humidity dermatoses. Occupational exposure to ozone may also occur in ultraviolet (UV)-curing processes, in the printing industry and during welding operations.

See also 'Arc welding of metal' (page 13).

Chapter 3

Fumes, fires and other environmental emissions

(a) Exposures during welding

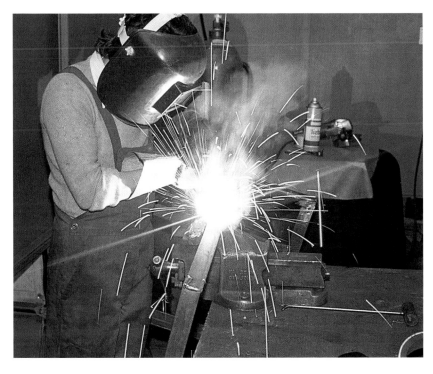

Figure 3.1 Arc welding of metal. Copyright Margaret Anne Harrison. Reproduced with permission.

Measurements of exposure to respiratory hazards may be obtained by personal sampling at work. A pump draws air through a sampling head, which is situated in the breathing zone. The illustrations show the correct positioning of the sampling head in the breathing zone.

Metal welding is the joining together of metals through the application of heat and sometimes also of local pressure. Classical welding processes produce fumes containing a mixture of gases and fine particles. The composition will depend on the welding process and the type of metal being joined. The metals being joined may be coated with other metals, such as zinc, lead, chromates or cadmium. In addition, halogen-containing solvents may have been used to clean the metal surfaces. The gases produced include oxides of nitrogen and ozone. Phosgene may be liberated if a solvent such as trichloroethylene is broken down by a welding flame. Respiratory effects due to welding may be irritation of the respiratory tract, metal fume fever and possible long-term respiratory impairment. Siderosis may be found in electric arc welders. It results from inhaling iron oxide in welding fume, usually after years of exposure, and may be associated with lung fibrosis. However, it is a matter of contention as to whether these conditions co-exist or whether siderosis may be a fibrogenic condition in some circumstances. Welding also exposes workers to electromagnetic radiation. Arc welding produces ultraviolet radiation, which may cause a severe conjunctivitis if the eyes are unshielded. UV(B) and UV(C) are absorbed by the conjunctiva, whereas UV(A) is absorbed mainly in the lens. Skin exposure to UV radiation may increase the risk of skin cancer.

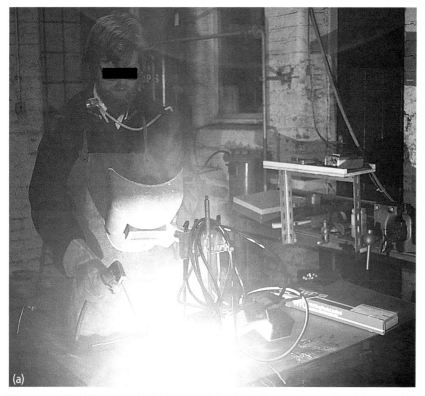

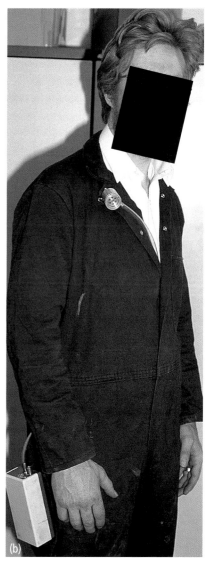

Figure 3.2 (a) Welding without local exhaust ventilation. (b) Monitoring equipment for welding. Copyright John Harrison. Reproduced with permission.

Risk assessment is fundamental to the control of risks in the workplace. Where possible, hazardous substances should be eliminated from work processes, or the processes modified, such as by removing the man from the process. The increasing sophistication of computer-controlled technology has made it possible for modern industrial plants, such as those involved in car manufacturing, to use robots to carry out welding. These machines are fast and accurate and do not develop industrial diseases. Local exhaust ventilation is included in the machinery to protect the general working environment, and access to the robots is strictly controlled, with interlock safety systems to ensure the segregation of workers from the moving robot.

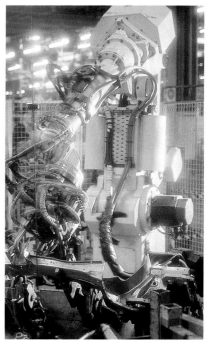

Figure 3.3 Welding robot body assembly. Reproduced courtesy of Nissan.

(b) Exposures during fires

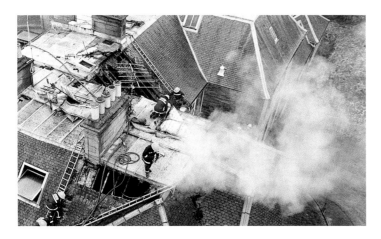

Figure 3.4 Fire officers exposed to smoke. Copyright Chris Ide. Reproduced with permission.

Fires cause the production of smoke and a range of toxic gases, as well as heat and oxygen deficiency. The products of combustion (or pyrolysis) will vary according to the prevailing conditions in the fire, such as the amount of oxygen, the temperature and the materials being burnt. Typical constituents of smoke include:

- soot
- carbon monoxide
- carbon dioxide
- nitrogen oxides
- hydrogen cyanide
- hydrogen chloride
- sulphur dioxide
- hydrogen fluoride

- hydrogen sulphide
- isocyanates
- acrolein
- benzene
- phenol
- formaldehyde
- chlorinated hydrocarbons.

Inhalation of carbon monoxide is said to be an important factor in 50–80 per cent of fatalities due to fire.

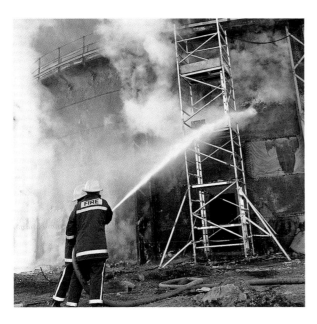

Figure 3.5 Major hazard emergencies: fire officers attending a fire at a water tank. Copyright Chris Ide. Reproduced with permission.

Fires at industrial sites are of particular concern. Apart from the fire itself and its inherent dangers, there is the possibility of an explosion or a major release of toxic gas. Legislation was introduced in many European countries following an incident in Italy when dioxin was released over a wide area near Seveso and 178 children developed chloracne. The owners of chemical sites are required to assess the risks of the on-site and off-site release of dangerous substances, to control risks to both people and the environment, and to have detailed agreed emergency plans accessible to the emergency services. If such an incident does occur, all emergency services are usually involved and this requires careful co-ordination and excellent communication.

(c) Controlling and monitoring environmental emissions

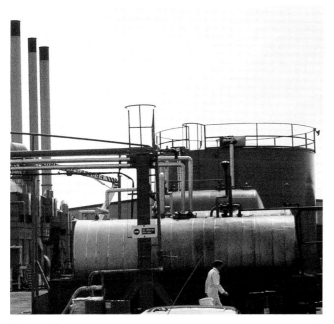

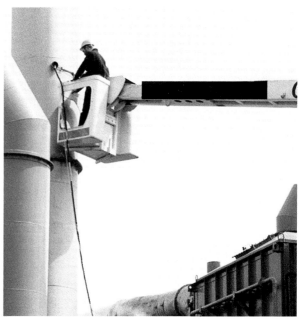

Figure 3.6 Modern emission stacks. Copyright John Harrison. Reproduced with permission.

Figure 3.7 Measuring emissions from a mobile platform. Copyright John Harrison. Reproduced with permission.

Environmental legislation places duties on companies to reduce environmental emissions. Emissions from stacks may be monitored using different techniques, according to the type of emission. Isokinetic sampling is used to measure particulates and for volatile organic chemicals an analyser involving a flame-ionization detection process is the method of choice. Companies must provide safe access for measurements to be made and should consider the need for monitoring in the design of new plant. For existing plant, a mobile platform may still be necessary for access.

Chapter 4 | Pesticides and other agrochemicals

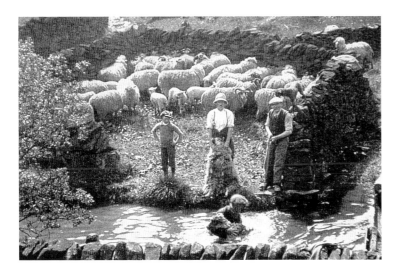

Figure 4.1 Historical sheep dipping. Copyright Margaret Anne Harrison. Reproduced with permission.

Modern sheep dips contain organophosphate pesticides. Earlier dips contained arsenic compounds and were also dangerous to the farmers. Today, arsenic exposure may occur, in addition, in smelting and in the chemical, pesticide and pharmaceutical industries. The gas arsine is also used in the electronics industry. Arsenic may cause acute or chronic poisoning. Acute poisoning following ingestion presents as abdominal pain, vomiting, rice water stools, dehydration and shock. Chronic poisoning may cause dermatitis, ulceration, hyperkeratosis of the palms and soles and raindrop pigmentation of the skin. Skin cancer has been described in sheep dippers. A mixed peripheral neuropathy due to interference with glycolysis in neurons may develop, which may respond to British Anti-Lewisite (BAL; dimercaprol). Hepatic cirrhosis and megaloblastic anaemia are associated with chronic arsenic exposure, as is the perforation of the cartilaginous nasal septum. Health surveillance by measuring urinary arsenic, monomethyl arsonic acid and cacodylic acid gives an estimate of recent exposures.

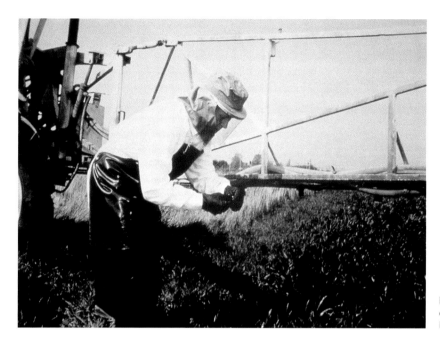

Figure 4.2 Man preparing for automated spraying of pesticides onto crops. Copyright Margaret Anne Harrison. Reproduced with permission.

Pesticides are preparations used to control or destroy organisms that interfere with agriculture, horticulture or the environment. The types of chemicals used are organophosphates, carbamates and organochlorine compounds. Many of these are absorbed into the body by inhalation or through the skin and can cause severe ill-health effects. Consequently, it is essential for workers spraying pesticides to wear the correct protective clothing and respiratory protection. Health surveillance and biological monitoring are usually required and may be statutory obligations. Organophosphates and carbamates are cholinesterase inhibitors. However, the latter cause short-lived inhibition and the use of oxime antidotes is not recommended. The activity of acetyl cholinesterase is genetically determined and about 4 per cent of UK, French and American individuals have reduced levels of activity compared to the general population. This renders them more susceptible to toxicity from organophosphates. Organochlorine compounds include pentachlorophenol (PCP) and dichlorodiphenyltrichloroethane (DDT). PCP causes mucosal irritation, respiratory and neurological disturbances. There may also be hyperpyrexia. Chloracne has been described in woodworkers. DDT causes central nervous system effects and hepatic damage. Concerns about its persistence in the food chain have led to its withdrawal from general use.

See also 'Chloracne' (page 101).

Chapter 5 | Aliphatic and aromatic chemicals

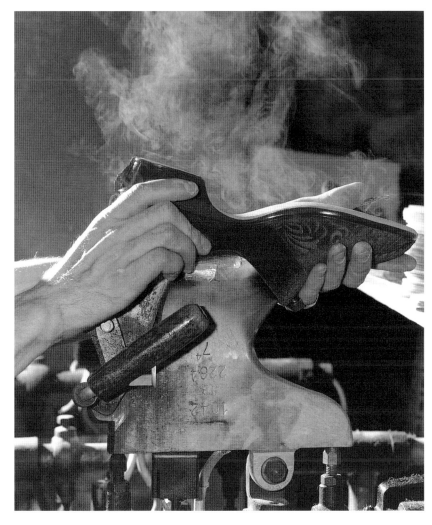

Figure 5.1 Solvent fume exposure in shoe manufacturing. Copyright Health & Safety Laboratory, Sheffield, UK. Reproduced with permission.

Solvents and glues are used to fix the sole to the top of a shoe. They are usually volatile and give off fumes in increased amounts if warmed. Solvent inhalation produces symptoms of central nervous system (CNS) depression such as fatigue and drowsiness. Specific solvents such as n-hexane may result in damage to peripheral nerves producing neuropathy.

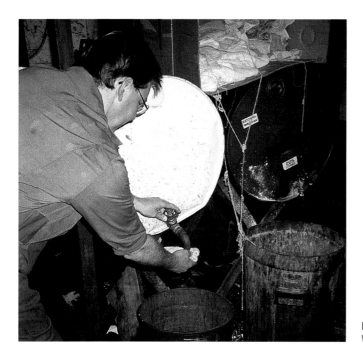

Figure 5.2 Dermal exposure to solvents in plating. Copyright Nerys R. Williams. Reproduced with permission.

The principal occupational skin irritants are soaps, detergents and organic solvents. The protective superficial layer of the epidermis is comprised of a very thin lipoprotein membrane. Continual exposure to skin irritants leads to a defatting of the superficial skin barrier, which makes the skin more vulnerable to damage from trauma and to the action of the various chemicals that might come into contact with it. Contact irritant dermatitis results when chemicals capable of causing cell damage are applied for sufficient time and in sufficient concentration. An example of an organic solvent that is used widely in industry as a metal degreaser is trichloroethylene ('trike'). It has been estimated that as many as 10 000 degreasing units exist in the UK. Trichloroethylene is readily absorbed through the skin, although the principal route of absorption is via inhalation. Ill-health effects include CNS disturbances, narcosis and possible death. Facial nerve palsy and peripheral mononeuropathies have been reported. Sudden death, possibly as a result of ventricular fibrillation, may occur. Less severe, but also disturbing, is the occurrence of 'degreasers' flush' (pronounced facial blushing) in workers who drink alcohol after working with the solvent.

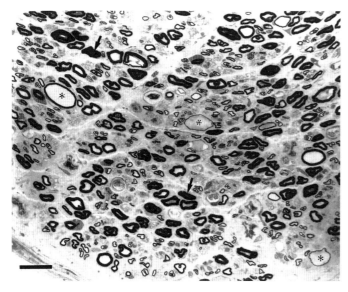

Figure 5.3 Sural nerve biopsy showing neuropathy related to solvent exposure (bar – 20 μm). Copyright P.K. Thomas. Reproduced with permission.

The illustration shows a transverse section through a sural nerve biopsy specimen from a subject with giant axonal neuropathy related to exposure to industrial solvent. Enlarged axons surrounded by thin myelin are indicated by asterisks. In other fibres (arrowed), the axons are shrunken so that the surrounding myelin sheath has collapsed.

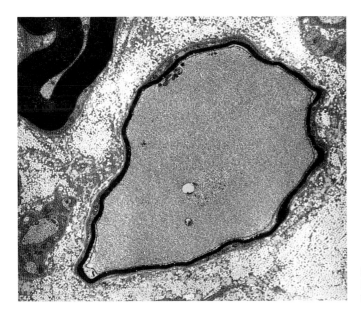

Figure 5.4 Electron micrograph of nerve biopsy showing effects of industrial solvent exposure (bar – 1 µm). Copyright P.K. Thomas. Reproduced with permission.

This figure is an electron micrograph from a nerve biopsy from a subject exposed to industrial solvent showing a 'giant axon' filled with neurofilaments and surrounded by an abnormally thin myelin sheath. A portion of a fibre with a shrunken axon and surrounded by a collapsed myelin sheath is seen in the upper left corner.

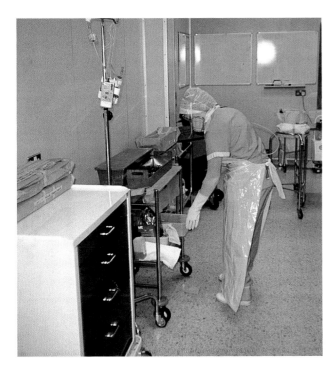

Figure 5.5 Use of glutaraldehyde in the sterilization of endoscopy equipment. Copyright Ian R. Gardner, Health & Safety Executive, UK. Reproduced with permission.

Within the hospital and healthcare settings, particularly endoscopy suites, glutaraldehyde is used as a very effective cold sterilizer of medical equipment that cannot be autoclaved. Unfortunately, it is also a common skin irritant and cases of occupational asthma have been reported in hospital staff. The mechanism of causation of the asthma is not clear – IgE antibodies are not found in the blood and the asthma may be due to either sensitization or irritation. Rhinitis and conjunctivitis may also be reported. Control of exposure is achieved by the use of less harmful agents, enclosure and local exhaust ventilation. Residual risk is controlled by the use of gloves, masks and glasses and by health surveillance.

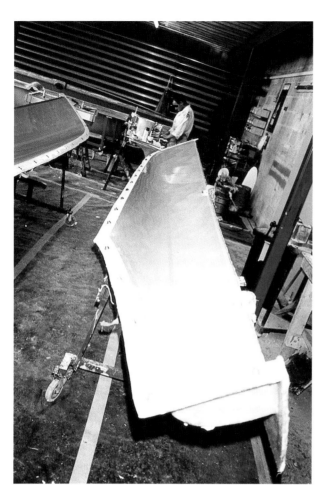

Figure 5.6 Styrene exposure during boat building. Copyright Paul Roberts. Reproduced with permission.

The manufacture of glass-reinforced plastic baths and boats uses styrene, a colourless solvent present in a resin that evaporates from between layers of fibrous glass. The gas enters the body via the lungs (entry through the skin is not significant), is metabolized in the liver via the cytochrome P450 system and is excreted as mandelic (up to 90 per cent) and phenylglyoxalic acids (up to 10 per cent). The measurement of these acids can be used for biological monitoring, although the consumption of alcohol produces spuriously low levels in exposed workers.

Acute exposure above 100 ppm causes irritation of the eyes and mouth, drowsiness and nausea. It is not clear whether lower level exposures have a significant effect on individuals, as although some studies have shown effects on psychomotor functioning, the exact significance of these findings is not clear. The World Health Organization's International Agency for Research on Cancer (IARC) has classified the agent as a group 2 possible human carcinogen.

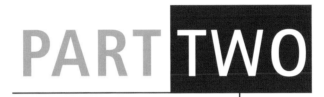

PART TWO

DISEASES ASSOCIATED WITH PHYSICAL AGENTS

6 Sound, noise and the ear

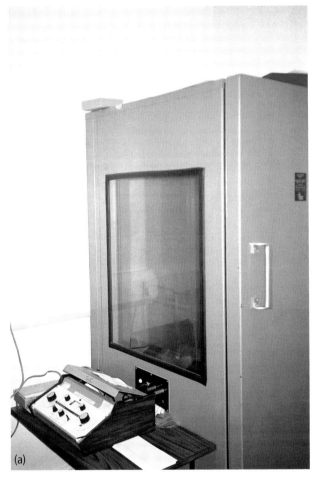
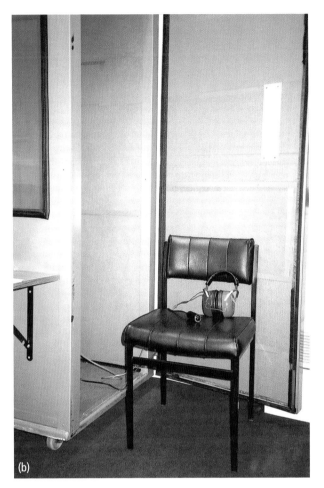

Figure 6.1 Audiometry equipment: (a) audiometer and booth; (b) headphones and booth door, insulated against external noise. Copyright John Harrison. Reproduced with permission.

Audiometry is a useful procedure to detect hearing loss due to noise. It should be carried out in a booth to reduce background noise to levels of less than 5 decibels. Machines vary in their capabilities: the more sophisticated models calculate the hearing capability over a range of frequencies and calculate any hearing loss. Results are then presented according to a system published in a draft document by the UK Health and Safety Executive (HSE) entitled *Audiometry in Industry*. Older models, such as the one shown, require manual calculation of hearing loss.

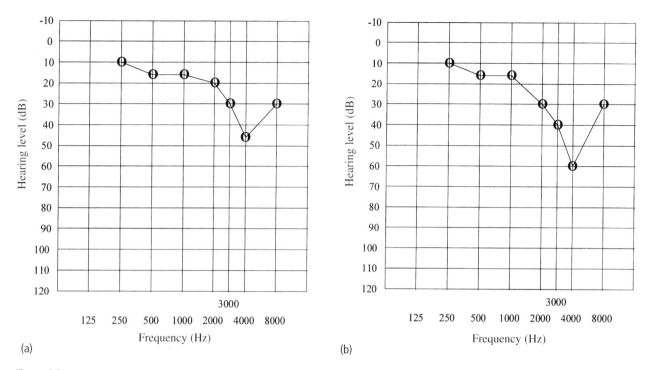

Figure 6.2 Pure tone audiograms – right ear – showing (a) the typical 4 kHz notch after excessive noise exposure; (b) a deepening of the 4 kHz notch and involvement of adjacent frequencies. Reproduced from *Hunter's Diseases of Occupations*, 9th edition, edited by P.J. Baxter, P.H. Adams, T.C. Aw, A. Cockcroft and J.M. Harrington, published in 2000 by Arnold with permission of R.T. Ramsden.

Noise-induced deafness produces a classic pattern of a reduction in hearing at the 4 kHz range, which can be seen as a characteristic dip at 4 kHz on the trace. This loss of hearing capability falls within the normal range of speech and is severely disabling. In addition to noise exposure, similar patterns of hearing loss can occur due to toxins such as alcohol, quinine and carbon disulphide, and in syphilis, cerebral contusion and the deafness associated with retinitis pigmentosa. The pattern differs from that seen in age-related deafness or presbycusis, in which there is a gradual reduction in loss at all of the higher frequencies. It is important that audiometry is conducted in a sound-proof booth on individuals who have not been exposed to noise during the previous 48 hours. If the latter requirement is not met, the individual may show a pattern of the phenomenon of temporary threshold shift, which is a reversible loss of hearing at 4 kHz.

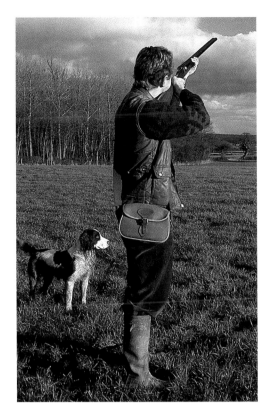

Figure 6.3 Unilateral noise exposure from the use of a shotgun. Copyright Nerys R. Williams. Reproduced with permission.

Recreational shooting (either indoor or outdoor) without adequate hearing protection may lead to unilateral hearing loss. The loss occurs in the ear nearest to the side of ejection of the cartridge rather than the barrel of the gun. Usually occupational exposure in a noisy environment produces bilateral deafness with the classical 4 kHz notch on both sides. Typically noisy operations include those in foundries, industrial laundries, drop forges and engineering workshops.

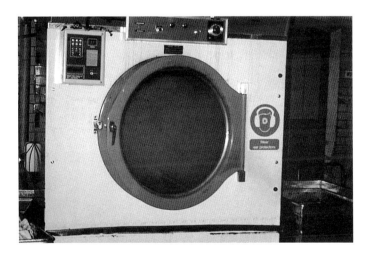

Figure 6.4 A commercial laundry machine. Copyright John Harrison. Reproduced with permission.

Noise is an important occupational hazard and occupational noise-induced damage to hearing is said to be one of the commonest occupational disorders in developed countries. The machines used in laundries are often noisy, with levels exceeding 85 dB(A) (the most commonly used weighted scale when measuring noise levels in the workplace). Employers are required to conduct risk assessments, measure noise levels and calculate exposures over a working day, and implement control measures. This may include ensuring the maintenance of equipment and the use of noise-absorbing materials and also providing health surveillance.

7 Vibration (hand–arm and whole body)

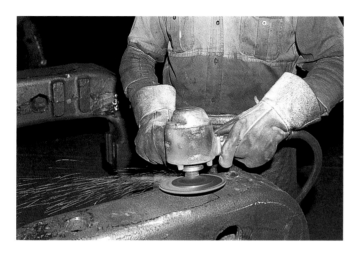

Figure 7.1 Hand-held air grinder used to smooth metal. Copyright Peter Pelmear. Reproduced with permission.

A number of hand-held tools may be associated with the development of the hand–arm vibration syndrome (HAVS). They include drills, guns (e.g. riveting gun), impact tools, grinders, sanders and saws. A variety of grinders generate vibration of sufficient severity and at frequencies that have the potential to increase the risk of the development of symptoms. The optimum frequencies for causing vasoconstriction are reported to be 30–60 Hz, 125 Hz or 125–500 Hz. In addition, exposure to cold – either because of working outdoors or because of the direction of cold exhaust air onto the hands – will increase the risk of symptoms. Prevention of the occurrence of the HAVS depends on reducing exposures by improving the design of hand-held tools. The reduction of vibration at source, followed by ensuring adequate damping and good ergonomic design to decrease hand pressures when using the tools, is the main aim. Wearing gloves does not provide sufficient attenuation of vibration to make this a reliable preventive measure, although it does help to keep the hands dry and to protect the skin from trauma. Ultimately, the automation of processes is likely to have the biggest impact on reducing the HAVS.

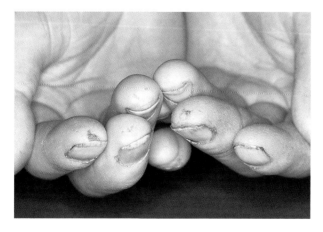

Figure 7.2 Clinical manifestations of hand–arm vibration syndrome. Copyright Peter Pelmear. Reproduced with permission.

The diagnosis of HAVS is based on obtaining a history of fingers blanching when exposed to the cold and of significant exposure to hand–arm vibration and the absence of another recognized cause of Raynaud's phenomenon. At present, the performance of additional objective tests may support the clinical diagnosis, but the finding of normal test results does not preclude a diagnosis of HAVS.

Cold water provocation tests have, until recently, been the standard method used to assess the vascular response to cold. There are several variations to the method, but the aim is to cool the fingers to a specified temperature, usually between 10°C and 15°C, and to measure changes in blood pressure, skin temperature or colour. Measurements are taken before, during and after cooling. Recent large-scale studies have, however, cast doubt on the sensitivity and specificity of this test. Finger systolic blood pressure (FSBP) following cooling of the fingers has been reported as having acceptable sensitivity and specificity for diagnosis, but is relatively expensive and technically difficult to perform. A typical trace arising from an FSBP test is shown below.

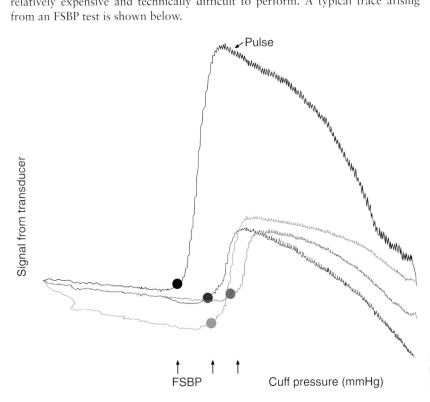

Figure 7.3 Finger systolic blood pressure tests for hand–arm vibration syndrome: a typical trace. Copyright Ian Lawson. Reproduced with permission.

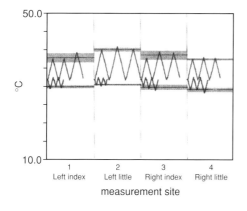

Site	Hot thrsh.	Cold thrsh.	Neutral zone
1	37.8°C	29.9°C	8.0°C
2	40.0°C	30.4°C	9.6°C
3	38.5°C	29.6°C	8.9°C
4	37.4°C	28.9°C	8.4°C

Normal thermogram

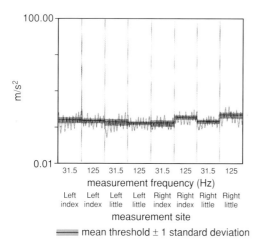

Frequency	Threshold
31.5 Hz	0.156 m/s^2
125.0 Hz	0.149 m/s^2
31.5 Hz	0.138 m/s^2
125.0 Hz	0.130 m/s^2
31.5 Hz	0.132 m/s^2
125.0 Hz	0.192 m/s^2
31.5 Hz	0.148 m/s^2
125.0 Hz	0.226 m/s^2

mean threshold ± 1 standard deviation

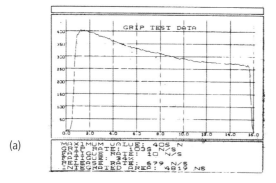

Figure 7.4 Results of sensorineural tests for hand–arm vibration syndrome: (a) normal. Copyright Ian Lawson. Reproduced with permission.

(a)

Normal grip strength profile

There are several tests of sensorineural function that may be used to assess the HAVS objectively. As in the case of cold water provocation tests, a positive result supports the clinical diagnosis of HAVS, but a negative result does not completely rule it out. However, some investigators believe that severe HAVS is unlikely to occur in the absence of positive sensorineural results from a battery of tests. A typical battery would include some or all of the following: vibration perception thresholds, thermal detection threshold tests and grip strength. Nerve conduction studies may also be used. Current perception threshold testing also appears to be

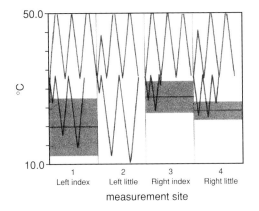

Site	Hot thrsh. —	Cold thrsh.—	Neutral zone
1	52.1°C	20.1°C	31.9°C
2	49.2°C	17.8°C	31.4°C
3	51.4°C	27.9°C	23.5°C
4	49.2°C	24.3°C	24.9°C

Abnormal thermogram
Increase in temperature
neutral zone (TNZ)

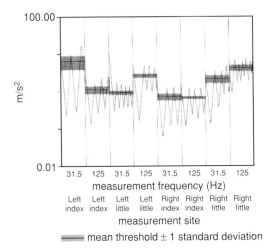

Frequency	Threshold
31.5 Hz	6.575 m/s^2
125.0 Hz	1.168 m/s^2
31.5 Hz	0.974 m/s^2
125.0 Hz	2.750 m/s^2
31.5 Hz	0.751 m/s^2
125.0 Hz	0.707 m/s^2
31.5 Hz	2.243 m/s^2
125.0 Hz	4.350 m/s^2

══════ mean threshold ± 1 standard deviation

Abnormal vibrogram

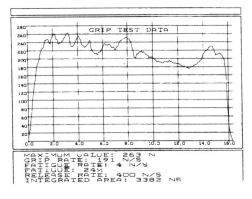

Grip strength profile of poor technique
or submaximal effort

(b)

Figure 7.4 (continued) Results of sensorineural tests for hand–arm vibration syndrome: (b) abnormal. Copyright Ian Lawson. Reproduced with permission.

gaining popularity. Vibrometers are used to measure vibration perception. Testing at 31.5 Hz and 125 Hz is recommended, although testing over a frequency range 8–500 Hz might be considered. Thermal detection involves placing the finger pulp on a metal plate, the temperature of which is varied. Testing is usually computer controlled. Hot and cold zones are defined, as well as the difference between them. Grip strength is measured with a dynamometer. The best of two or more flexor contractions is usually recorded for each wrist. For all these tests, good normative data are required for comparison.

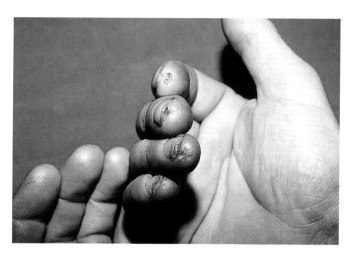

Figure 7.5 Digital gangrene due to vibration exposure. Copyright Peter Pelmear. Reproduced with permission.

Digital vasospasm associated with exposure to hand–arm vibration is a recognized condition. Trophic changes at the fingertips, although rare, may occur if there is prolonged and severe exposure to hand–arm vibration and associated risks of trauma and cold. Pathological studies of digital vessels exposed to vibration have demonstrated muscular hypertrophy and intimal fibrosis. The latter is more likely in severe cases. The release of chemical vasodilators and vasoconstrictors from the endothelium may be important following vessel wall injury or endothelial damage. Vasospasm may also occur in primary Raynaud's disease and in scleroderma, which has been associated with exposure to vibration, silica, vinyl chloride monomer and a variety of other substances. The severity of cold-induced Raynaud's phenomenon in the HAVS may be graded using the Stockholm Workshop scale. The most severe, grade 4, is characterized by frequent attacks of blanching of the fingers, affecting all phalanges of most of the fingers, with the presence of trophic changes.

Chapter 8   Heat and cold

(a) Heat exposure in the workplace

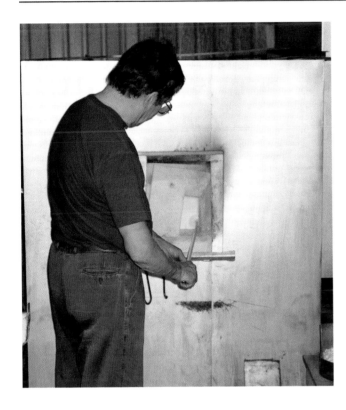

Figure 8.1 Heat exposure at a glass furnace prior to blowing. Copyright Nerys R. Williams. Reproduced with permission.

Close proximity to furnaces occurs in a variety of settings, such as foundries and glass works. Furnaces emit very high radiant heat, which may rarely cause cataracts in the eyes. Far more commonly, workers may complain of heat fatigue and heat stress, especially when external ambient temperatures are raised, such as in the summer. The prevention of heat-induced illness includes shielding workers from the heat source, increasing the distance from the furnace face to the worker, providing protective clothing that allows reflection of the heat and does not cause overheating of the body and, finally, ensuring adequate fluid intake and rest breaks. Working in hot environments is particularly likely to cause ill-health when it is also associated with heavy physical exertion. In such cases, ergonomic assessments and measurement of the thermal environment are essential.

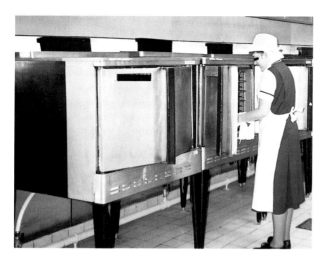

Figure 8.2 Exposure to radiant heat in the workplace: kitchen assistant unloading a commercial oven. Copyright John Harrison. Reproduced with permission.

Workers in close proximity to radiant heat sources, such as commercial ovens and laundries, are at risk of developing heat stress, particularly during the summer months when the ambient room temperature is likely to be uncomfortably high. Dry bulb temperature is only one measurement of the thermal climate that can be used to assess the conditions. Most measures of heat stress combine measurements of dry bulb temperature, humidity, radiant temperature and air velocity. A simple index that may be used in hot environments is the wet bulb globe temperature (WBGT) index. This requires measurement of the dry bulb temperature, wet bulb temperature and globe temperature, and estimates radiant temperature. An alternative index is the corrected effective temperature. For assessing indoor office environments, Fanger (1973) has produced two indices: Predicted Mean Vote (PMV) and Predicted Percentage Dissatisfied (PPD), based on a derived comfort equation. These indices take into account metabolic rate and clothing insulation, in addition to the four environmental parameters of thermal comfort.

Occupational heat exposure occurs in the outdoor environment of workers in hot countries, across a range of industrial sectors including leisure and tourism. Lifeguards at outdoor swimming pools and beach towers are exposed not only to high ambient temperatures, but also to sunlight, which may cause sunburn and skin cancers. The radiant and reflected heat may cause fatigue, heat stress and heat exhaustion. The combined effect of the temperature and the ergonomic demands of the task of the lifeguard (i.e. the need for observation and concentration), the reflection of the sun on water and the low likelihood of the need for an emergency response limit the periods of time that should be spent in one location before rotating and then resting. Other preventive strategies include sheltered seating and adequate hydration.

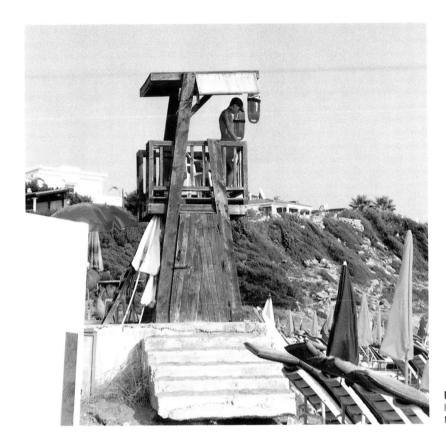

Figure 8.3 Environmental exposure to heat and UV light: lifeguard on duty, Coral Bay, Cyprus. Copyright Nerys R. Williams. Reproduced with permission.

(b) Cold exposure in the workplace

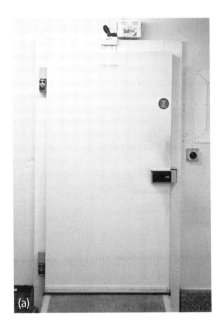
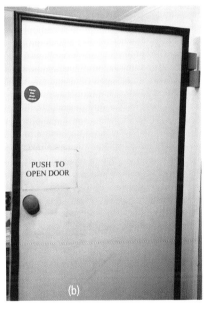

PUSH TO
OPEN DOOR

(a)

(b)

Figure 8.4 Commercial food freezer: (a) view from the outside; (b) view from the inside, showing dead man's handle to facilitate escape. Copyright John Harrison. Reproduced with permission.

Many commercial or public catering establishments have large freezers for storing food or foodstuffs. Cook–chill has become popular, whereby food is prepared and cooked centrally, chilled and distributed to peripheral food outlets. The temperature inside a freezer such as the one shown may be $-18°C$. Exposure to temperatures below $0°C$ without protection will cause local freezing of the tissues. Reduction in the body core temperature may occur if the exposure to such temperatures is prolonged. The selection of personal protective equipment against cold must take into account loss of manual dexterity. The accumulation of perspiration may become a problem if the clothing is worn for prolonged periods. This reduces the level of insulation. There should be rules guarding against people working alone in walk-in freezers and there should be a dead-man's handle on the inside of the door to prevent workers becoming trapped inside.

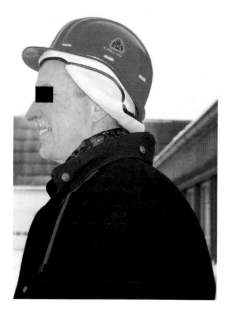

Figure 8.5 Personal protective equipment for working in extremes of low temperature: fur-lined ear covers worn under a hard hat. Copyright Nerys R. Williams. Reproduced with permission.

Work outside in extremes of temperature may require the use of specialized personal protective equipment (PPE). The slide shows a worker wearing fur ear covers under a hard hat while working at a foundry in Northern Finland. Temperatures of 20°C below freezing are common outside the main buildings which workers cross between.

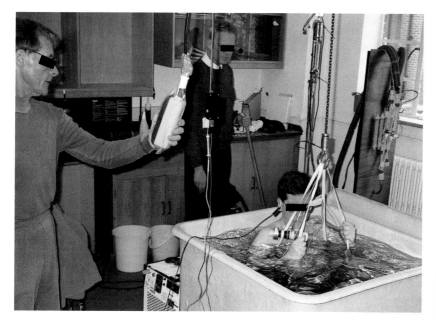

Figure 8.6 Clinical evaluation of the effects on the human body of immersion in cold water. Copyright Peter Blain and Reza Hossain. Reproduced with permission from Peter Blain.

The physiological responses to immersion in cold water include hyperventilation, tachycardia and vasoconstriction. Repeated brief exposures to cold can produce adaptation to these responses (habituation). The degree of hyperventilation and tachycardia may be attenuated by such exposures. It has been suggested that cold adaptation may confer an advantage on workers who are required to spend time in cold climates, permitting sleep and greater comfort. It is less clear whether such immersions confer an advantage during the later stages of cold exposure. Earlier and marked cold vasodilatation is another change that has been reported in association with prolonged exposure to cold, e.g. in fish filleters.

Reference

P.O. Fanger, *Thermal Comfort*. McGraw-Hill, *New York*, 1973.

Chapter 9

Raised barometric pressure: diving

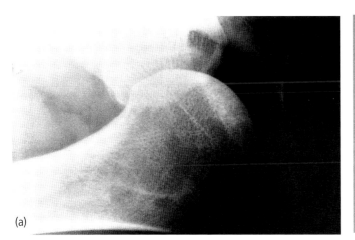 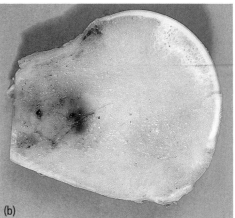

Figure 9.1 (a) X-ray of shoulder joint. (b) Pathological section through head of humerus. Copyright Joe Pooley. Reproduced with permission.

Dysbaric osteonecrosis used to be a crippling complication of long-term exposures to raised environmental pressure during commercial diving. The first cases of bone necrosis presented in people working with compressed air involving tunnelling, a technique of excavating in wet locations. There is a statistical relationship between the occurrence of the 'bends' and the development of dysbaric osteonecrosis, but the association is a weak one. There is evidence that saturation dives are more likely to cause necrosis than short dives to less than 30 metres. There are two main types of lesion, according to the Medical Research Council radiological classification: subchondral lesions (or A lesions) and lesions in the heads of long bones (B lesions). The development of A lesions may be a precursor to the occurrence of juxta-articular lesions. Consequently, such findings on screening have been used as the basis for advice to divers to cease further exposures to raised environmental pressures. The incidence of abnormal findings on routine x-ray screening of the long bones of commercial divers has decreased in recent times, such that this investigation is no longer performed annually.

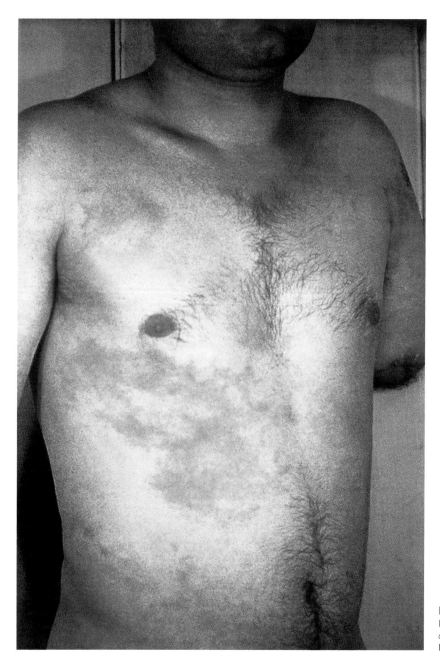

Figure 9.2 Skin lesions of decompression sickness. Reproduced with permission from *Diving and Subaquatic Medicine*, 4th edition, C. Edmonds, C. Lowry, J. Pennefather & R. Walker. Arnold, London, 2002.

Decompression illness is thought to occur in association with the evolution of bubbles in the body, as gases that had dissolved in tissues whilst under increased pressure are released. Thus, the occurrence of decompression illness requires a sufficient stay at a depth of water to allow gas uptake. Cutaneous decompression illness may manifest as itching in exposed parts or the development of a blotchy red or purple rash. A lymphatic form of illness may present as peau d'orange in the limbs or as oedema in the face or on the trunk. The occurrence of skin symptoms or signs is a warning that other, more serious, manifestations of decompression illness might occur. Divers with a rash are considered to be candidates for recompression treatment.

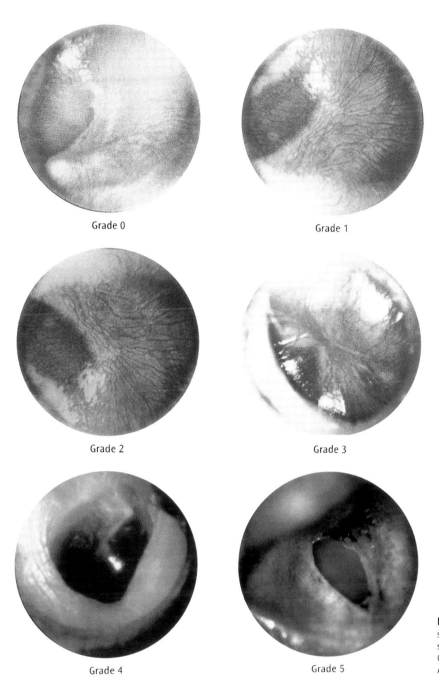

Grade 0

Grade 1

Grade 2

Grade 3

Grade 4

Grade 5

Figure 9.3 Middle-ear barotraumas of differing severity, graded by otoscopy. Reproduced with permission from *Diving and Sub-aquatic Medicine*, 4th edition, C. Edmonds, C. Lowry, J. Pennefather & R. Walker. Arnold, London, 2002.

All the anatomical sections of the ear may be affected by barotrauma. The key to protecting the middle ear from damage is a patent Eustachian tube, which allows equilibration of gas pressures between the middle ear and the external environment. Inability to 'clear the ears' may lead to middle ear barotrauma of varying severity. The mildest form is associated with some injection of vessels on the tympanic membrane. In more severe cases the degree of injection is marked and may be accompanied by a serosanguinous transudate; there may be rupture of the tympanic membrane. This condition is painful and may be accompanied by vertigo if cold water enters the middle ear following rupture of the membrane. Moderate and severe cases are treated with antibiotics and a return to diving is postponed until recovery has been achieved.

Chapter 10 Reduced barometric pressure: working at high altitude

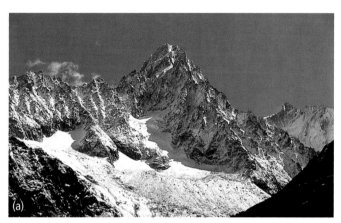 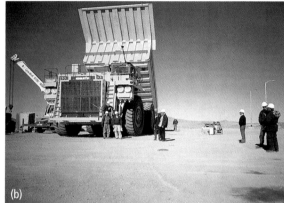

Figure 10.1 Working at high altitude: (a) mountains, (b) mining copper ore at altitude, Collahuasi mine, north Chile. (a) Copyright Nerys R. Williams. Reproduced with permission. (b) Copyright John B. West. Reproduced with permission.

When working at high altitude for periods long enough to allow acclimatization, e.g. copper mining in Chile, some people can achieve acclimatization in about a week. However, there is great variability. Past experience is a good guide to future performance.

Business travellers to countries such as Peru or Chile may not allow for the need to acclimatize, and experience the equivalent of hypoxia as they ascend. The fall in barometric pressure leads to a reduced partial pressure of oxygen in air and of arterial pO_2 and stimulation of ventilation. Within 1–2 days of arrival, they may develop symptoms of acute mountain sickness, feeling light headed, breathless and lethargic. The symptoms usually resolve over a further 1–2 days but in a small number of cases progress to pulmonary and then cerebral oedema. Travellers need guidance on prevention, including staging ascents where possible, the use of medication and the early identification of symptoms. Travellers with sickle cell anaemia need particularly careful evaluation prior to departure.

Chapter 11 Reduced atmospheric pressure: flying

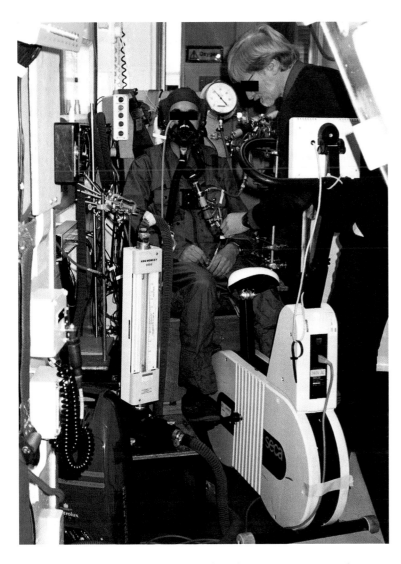

Figure 11.1 Experimental exposure to a hypobaric environment. Copyright Peter Blain and Reza Hossain. Reproduced with permission from Peter Blain.

Modern aviation involves exposure to hypobaric environments. This is true particularly for military aircrew. Reduction in atmospheric pressure causes hypoxia because the partial pressure of oxygen (pO_2) in the inspired air is reduced. The pO_2 cannot be allowed to fall below the critical level of 60 mmHg in the alveoli. At a height of 8000 feet (approximately 2500 m), the speed of reactions and learning ability have been shown to be impaired significantly. This is the maximum effective altitude for commercial aircraft. Many airforces stipulate that supplementary oxygen must be used when the cabin altitude exceeds 10 000 feet (approximately 3000 m). The hypobaric chamber is used to simulate flying at higher altitudes and to test breathing apparatus. Exercise physiology tested under such conditions can give important information about how the body reacts to extreme altitudes and can be used to test air supply systems.

Chapter 12 Ionizing radiations

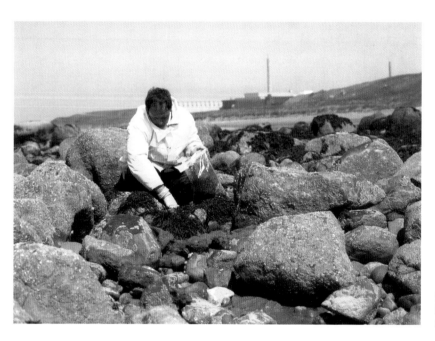

Figure 12.1 Environmental monitoring near the Sellafield Site. Copyright BNFL. Reproduced with permission.

Monitoring for ionizing radiation may be undertaken in a variety of locations, using a variety of methods – personal and environmental. Personal monitoring of workers may be undertaken using film badges. Environmental measurements can be made with thermoluminescent devices or Geiger counters. Occupational exposures in the UK occur in medical x-ray units, the nuclear industry, engineering (non-destructive testing) or road building (measurements). They are carefully controlled under the auspices of a national organization – the National Radiological Protection Board – and in accordance with legislation. Environmental exposure to ionizing radiation may occur from the inhalation of radon gas.

Occupational exposures to high levels of ionizing radiation are rare. The biological effects of exposures begin at about 0.1 Sv, whereas 1 Sv may cause mild acute radiation sickness in some people; 10 Sv cause severe acute radiation sickness, with depression of blood cell counts and damage to the gastrointestinal mucosa. An exposure of 8 Sv will cause erythema of the skin within a few hours, leading to a more intense inflammatory response over the next 7–10 days. Higher doses will cause increasing levels of damage, with moist desquamation and possible superinfection or serious fluid and protein loss. Survival will depend on accessing appropriate medical care and whether other tissues or organs have been damaged during the accidental exposure. If there has been exposure to and possible ingestion of a non-sealed source of radiation, the total absorbed dose can be measured.

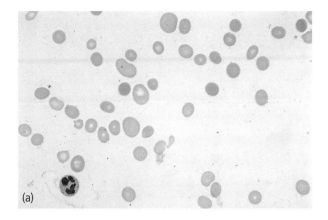

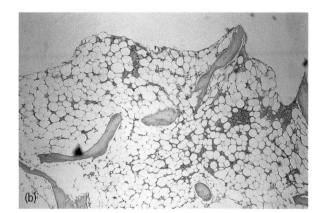

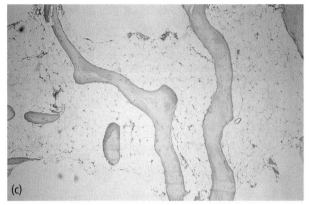

Figure 12.2 Bone marrow failure: (a) pancytopaenia; hypocellular marrow, (b) early, and (c) late. Copyright Jonathan Wallace. Reproduced with permission.

Bone marrow failure is an organ failure with a wide range of causes that exert their effect at different stages of blood cell development. This leads to a decrease in the numbers of circulating red cells, white cells and platelets. This is called pancytopaenia. Aplastic anaemia occurs when there is pancytopaenia and a hypocellular bone marrow and the cause is not readily identifiable, e.g. due to marrow infiltration. There are some well-recognized occupational causes of aplastic anaemia, such as benzene and ionizing radiation. It has been suggested that exposure to organic arsenicals or organochlorine compounds, such as lindane, might be associated with aplastic anaemia, but there is a lack of epidemiological evidence to support this.

Chapter 13 Non-ionizing radiation

The health risks resulting from exposure to microwaves, in communication workers, and from exposure to electromagnetic fields, in people working close to electrical appliances or power lines, have been a cause for concern. Microwave radiation is at the high-frequency end of the radio-frequency region of the electromagnetic spectrum. It has been suggested that exposure to microwave radiation may increase the risk of cataract formation, although animal experiments have failed to demonstrate this. Acute exposures to high levels of microwaves can cause skin burns and conjunctivitis. Other non-specific systemic symptoms have also been reported. Extremely low-frequency electric and magnetic fields have been linked to a raised incidence of tumours, such as leukaemia, brain cancer, breast cancer, lung cancer and malignant melanoma. There have also been reports of reproductive effects, such as congenital malformations. To date, none of these reports has been supported by studies that have accurate measures of radiation exposures. However, whether such exposures present a human health hazard remains controversial.

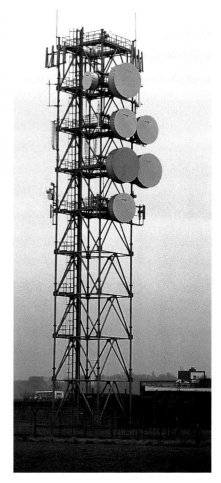

Figure 13.1 Mobile phone communication tower. Copyright D.L. Williams. Reproduced with permission.

PART THREE

DISEASES RELATED TO ERGONOMIC AND MECHANICAL FACTORS

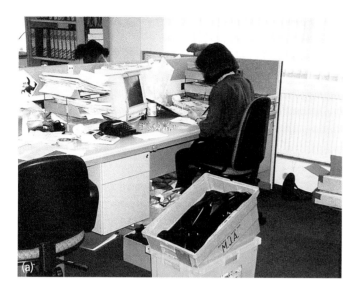

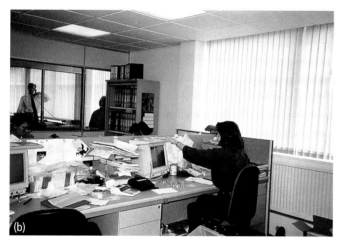

Figure 14.6 Worker using keyboard above monitor. Copyright Nerys R. Williams. Reproduced with permission.

Poor workstation design is a risk factor for the development of upper limb disorders. This worker had arranged her expensive new equipment to be used with the keyboard located on the top of the screen rather than on the desk. This was to enable her to sort small items directly in front of her to make up orders. Prolonged flexion of the shoulder in this abnormal non-physiological posture is likely to lead to complaints of pain and discomfort. The solution was to arrange her screen and work area so that the keyboard was operated with the arms at 90° at the elbows and the wrists moving at ±10° from the neutral position.

Chapter | *15* Back pain and work

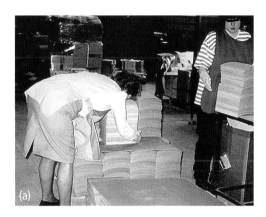
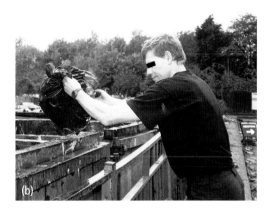

Figure 15.1 Poor posture during manual handling. (a) Copyright Peter Francis, Health & Safety Executive, Newcastle under Lyme, UK. Reproduced with permission. (b) Copyright Nerys R. Williams. Reproduced with permission.

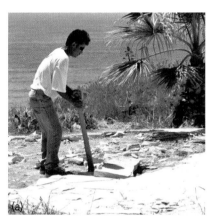
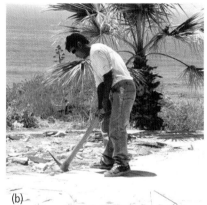
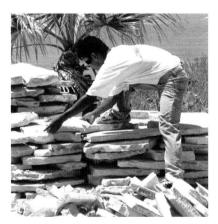
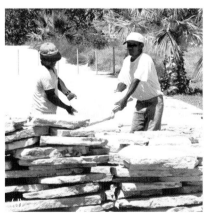

Figure 15.2 Manual handling in road building. (a) and (b) Flexion and use of pick. (c) Bending and lifting with poor stance. (d) Two-man lift, improved postures but rotation of lumber spine. Copyright Nerys R. Williams. Reproduced with permission.

The handling of loads may involve pushing and pulling as well as lifting. Risks of injury to the back or upper limbs are dependent not only on the weight lifted, but also on the posture needed for the lift. Lifting with the back outside of its normal range of movement places stresses on the soft and bony tissues of the spine. The majority of injuries to the back are due to damage to the soft tissues rather than the intervertebral discs, but the symptoms of pain, restriction of movement and disability are the same. Prevention of injury involves eliminating or modifying tasks, and providing lifting aids and training in safe lifting techniques.

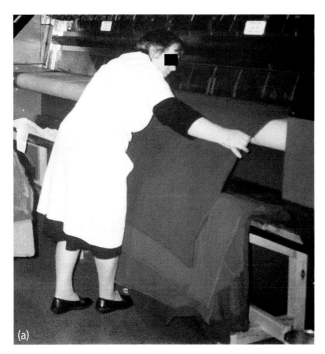 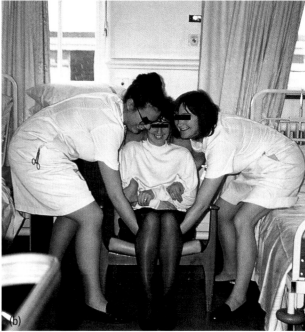

Figure 15.3 Low back pain. (a) Static stretching posture in a hospital laundry. (b) Manual handling: two nurses lifting a patient out of a chair in a hospital setting. Copyright John Harrison. Reproduced with permission.

Low back pain is common in the general population, and is a common symptom in workers whose jobs involve manual handling. Although the aetiology of back pain is complex, studies have shown that repetitive overuse and postural factors resulting from systems of work are associated with increased prevalence rates. It is not merely a requirement to lift heavy loads in jobs that leads to an increased risk of back pain; the prolonged maintenance of abnormal postures also causes marked increases in pressures on the spine because of the protective responses of the supporting muscles (see illustration a). Consequently, guidelines on manual handling should not merely focus on weights to be lifted, but should also include an assessment of the associated ergonomics.

In hospitals, the transfer of patients from a bed to a chair is a high-risk activity because of the poor ergonomics and cramped working environment (see figure b). Regulations require employers to minimize the risks to workers by avoiding lifting and handling manoeuvres except where they are unavoidable. The use of lifting aids and the provision of training are both important risk-reducing measures. All member states of the European Union have been required to implement the European directive on manual handling. There is increasing evidence that psychological risk factors are also important with respect to both the development of low back pain and the occurrence of chronic low back pain. The identification of these risk factors is a necessary component of a holistic risk assessment.

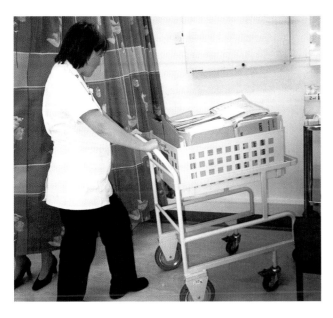

Figure 15.4 Manual handling in pregnancy: healthcare worker pushing a notes trolley in the outpatient department. Copyright Nerys R. Williams. Reproduced with permission.

A number of studies have looked at the risk to the mother and foetus from physically tiring work and strenuous exercise. The former has a reported association with amenorrhoea, and the latter may lead to an increased risk of abortion, stillbirth and foetal growth retardation. In the UK, it is a legal requirement for the work activities of pregnant or nursing mothers to be assessed specifically and all risks considered and reduced. The ergonomic aspects of the developing pregnancy and the resulting reduced flexibility and movement also need to be taken into account when assessing the job, and different recommendations may be appropriate at different stages of the pregnancy.

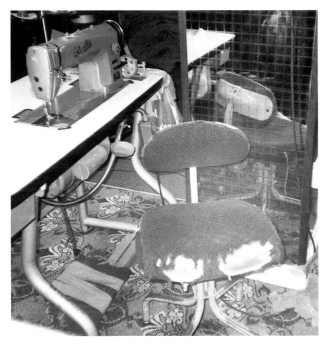

Figure 15.5 Inappropriate workplace seating in the textile industry: a risk factor for back pain. Copyright Nerys R. Williams. Reproduced with permission.

One area of the workplace environment that is often neglected, particularly in manufacturing industries, is seating. Standards exist in the office environment for display screen equipment users, but outside office environments seating is often not selected specifically for the task at hand. Seats need to be adjustable in height, with a foot rest either integral or separate, should provide adequate support to the back and should not apply pressure to the back of the knees. It is important that the cushion area remains intact to provide a comfortable surface for seating and that it avoids revealing any underlying hard metal or sharp surfaces. Ideally, seats should be personal to the individual worker and move with him or her where necessary, but where this is not possible, adjustable seating should be provided at every workstation.

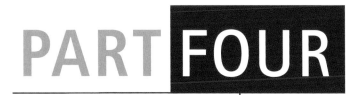

PART FOUR

DISEASES ASSOCIATED WITH MICROBIOLOGICAL AGENTS

(a) Amoebic dysentery

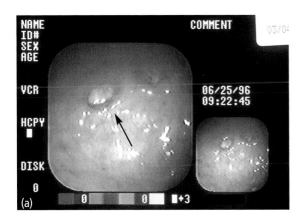

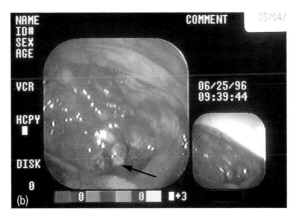

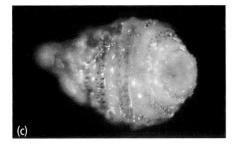

Figure 16.1 Amoebic ulceration (arrowed) of bowel mucosa. Copyright M.H. Snow. Reproduced with permission.

Enterotoxin-producing strains of *Escherichia coli* (ETEC) are the commonest cause of diarrhoea in travellers to less developed countries. Travellers who suffer from bloody diarrhoea should seek medical advice. *Entamoeba histolytica* is the cause of amoebic dysentery. Dysentery, the passage of loose stools containing fresh blood, occurs when there is generalized colonic ulceration or when there are lesions in the rectum or sigmoid colon. *Entamoeba histolytica* may exist as an intraluminal commensal in humans or it may invade the colonic mucosa. The pathological lesion is a lytic tissue necrosis. Sometimes the muscle coat of the colon may be breached, leading to intestinal perforation. The sites of ulceration are usually the rectosigmoid colon and caecum, but the entire colon may be involved. Hence the clinical manifestations may vary considerably. Abdominal tenderness and low-grade fever are common and hepatomegaly may be found if the ulceration is generalized. Stool microscopy usually shows large trophozoites, many containing ingested red blood cells (haematophagous). Sigmoidoscopy may be necessary in the absence of trophozoites in the stools.

Metronidazole is an effective treatment in short courses, although leucopenia or peripheral neuropathy may develop if it is used for a prolonged period. Emetine is a potent, but toxic, amoebicide. Dehydroemetine is a less toxic alternative. Chloroquine may be used to prevent hepatic lesions. The risk of acquiring amoebic dysentery is greatest in tropical and developing countries. Visitors to these countries should follow the instructions for simple basic hygiene: boiling water for 5 minutes, avoiding purchasing cooked foods from street stalls, eating only fruit that can be peeled and not eating salads that have been washed in untreated water. Food handlers who have suffered diarrhoea after a trip abroad should consult their occupational health department.

(b) Anthrax

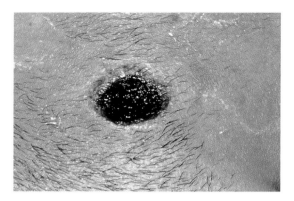

Figure 16.2 Cutaneous anthrax. Supplied by E. Gillanders, copyright R. Ian McCallum. Reproduced with permission.

Anthrax is a zoonotic disease caused by the Gram-positive organism *Bacillus anthracis*. It occurs in both animals and humans and in the latter case exists in three forms: cutaneous, gastrointestinal and respiratory. Occupational exposure is reported most commonly in tanners, who develop skin lesions from handling infected hides. However, this is rare, with only one or two cases reported in the UK each year. Ninety-five per cent of cases of anthrax affect the skin, entry usually occurring via a cut or graze. After an incubation period of 1–5 days, a vesicle develops, then ruptures and forms a necrotic ulcer, over which a black scab (or eschar) develops. Two to three weeks after exposure, the scab separates, resulting in a characteristic scar. Over this time period there may also be accompanying symptoms of headache, fever and malaise. With prompt antibiotic treatment, the mortality from cutaneous anthrax is very low, as distinct from the respiratory form, which is very aggressive and often fatal. Anthrax remains a potent biological warfare weapon because of its dispersal in the environment, resistant spore formation and devastating effect when inhaled.

(c) Chlamydia

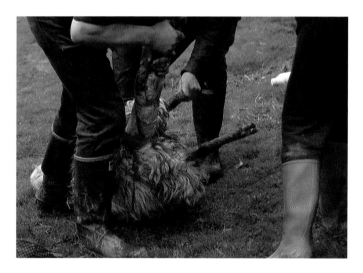

Figure 16.3 Lambing. Copyright D.G. Williams. Reproduced with permission.

Human infection with *Chlamydia psittaci* is associated with the development of psittacosis (see below). However, the same organism may also cause ovine enzootic abortion, or enzootic abortion of ewes. This infection is now known to have a worldwide distribution. Shepherdesses and farmers' wives may be exposed during the lambing season, and the peak incidence of the disease in sheep is between January and March in the UK. Infection is transmitted in fetal fluids and the placentae of infected sheep. However, serological testing of other farm workers has shown a widespread presence of antibodies to *Chlamydia*, suggesting that transmission is quite common but that infection is subclinical. Women who are pregnant are at particular risk of a clinical illness because of the presumed tropism of the *Chlamydia* for placental trophoblasts. A febrile illness, which may be severe, around lambing time should raise the possibility of infection and lead to treatment with antibiotics, such as erythromycin. Women farm workers who are, or who may be, pregnant should not participate in the lambing process.

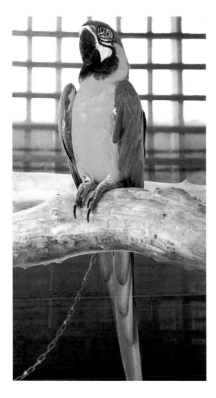

Figure 16.4 Psittacosis, a zoonosis acquired from parrots, is seen in bird handlers in pet shops, zoos and theme parks. Copyright Nerys R. Williams. Reproduced with permission.

Ornithosis is a zoonosis (an infection transmitted from animals to humans) acquired from birds infected with *Chlamydia psittaci*. When the infected birds come from the parrot family, the condition is known as psittacosis or 'parrot disease'. Cases usually arise from the keeping of pet birds, but outbreaks have been reported in flocks of chickens, turkeys and ducks. Domestic and wild pigeons are commonly affected and budgerigars have also been found to be a source of infection in Europe. Occupational groups at risk include pet shop owners, vets, poultry breeders, taxidermists, laboratory staff and construction workers. The infection is spread by inhalation, with symptoms of fever, headache and a flu-like illness. Pneumonia and endocarditis may follow. Treatment with antibiotics usually results in full recovery. Prevention is by the elimination of the organism from bird colonies, careful handling of birds to reduce dust, adequate ventilation in areas where birds are kept, and the use of appropriate personal protective equipment and work practices.

(d) Cowpox

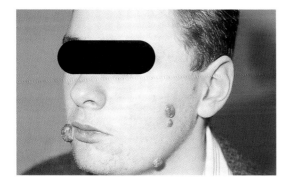

Figure 16.5 Cowpox in a vet. Copyright M.H. Snow. Reproduced with permission.

Cowpox has a place in history as the infection that led Edward Jenner to discover a successful vaccine against smallpox. Cowpox virus is a member of the poxviruses family and occupationally is likely to be spread by contact with cattle and cats. Only a few cases are reported each year in the UK, but those that do occur are found in laboratory staff, vets and herdsmen. Infection in humans usually produces a single lesion on the hands, forearms or face, which may be moderately severe. An inflamed local lesion is associated with regional adenopathy and systemic illness. Cowpox resolves in 4–6 weeks.

(e) Cutaneous larva migrans

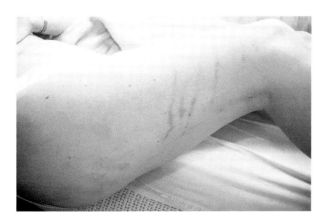

Figure 16.6   Cutaneous larva migrans. Copyright M.H. Snow. Reproduced with permission.

Helminths can be divided into roundworms, tapeworms and flukes. Helminthic infections are important causes of disease worldwide. In most cases, helminths cannot multiply in human hosts and the damage caused to the host is proportional to the worm burden. One exception to this rule is infection with *Strongyloides*. *Strongyloides stercoralis* may be found in the tropics and sub-tropics and people at most risk of infection are those who live or have lived in poor conditions in an endemic area. In the UK, it is known that ex-soldiers who were prisoners-of-war in the Far East could have become infected. Because of the ability of this type of worm to autoinfect its host, people remain infected and may die of fulminating disease many years after the initial infection. The worms develop in the duodenum and jejunum. Eggs or larvae are shed in the stools. Some larvae may become infective before they are shed in the stools and they penetrate the bowel wall and migrate to the lungs. In some situations, large numbers of larvae migrate, usually in cases of immunosuppression, diabetic ketoacidosis or other infections. The migration of larvae under the skin causes the development of urticarial wheals, producing a condition called cutaneous larva migrans. This condition, shown in the illustration affecting the leg of an anthropologist in South America, affects most chronically infected patients. The infection may be treated with ivermectin.

(f) HIV and hepatitis

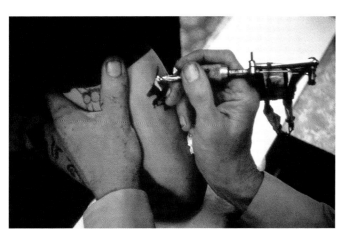

Figure 16.7   Unhygienic tattooing. Copyright Margaret Anne Harrison. Reproduced with permission.

Tattooing and body piercing are fashionable. There are important infection control issues associated with such activities, particularly the risk of transmission of blood-borne viruses. Outbreaks of hepatitis B have been traced back to tattoo parlours with poor standards of hygiene and infection control. Body piercing and some complementary health practices may also represent a risk. Hepatitis B is a highly infectious DNA-containing virus and the risk of infection following inoculation with hepatitis B e-antigen-positive material is approximately 30 per cent. Instruments that have been used for skin piercing must be autoclaved before they are re-used.

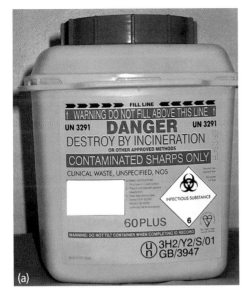

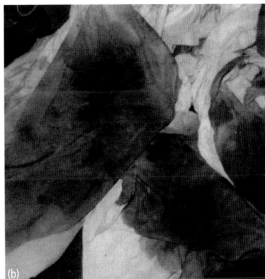

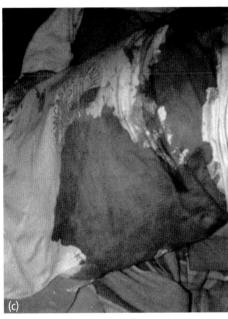

Figure 16.8 Sources of infection in hospitals: (a) sharps and needlestick injuries; (b) and (c) laundries. (a) Copyright Nerys R. Williams. Reproduced with permission. (b) and (c) – Copyright John Harrison. Reproduced with permission.

Sharps and needlestick injuries are relatively common in hospital settings, and are a documented transmission route for blood-borne infections such as human immunodeficiency virus (HIV) and hepatitis. Although much has been done to raise awareness of the importance of avoiding such injuries, a large hospital authority of about 10 000 employees might record 150 injuries per annum, but this is likely to represent gross under-reporting, particularly in surgery. Many of the reported injuries occur as a result of the careless disposal of needles, syringes, intravenous giving sets, lancets and operating instruments. The correct disposal of sharps is into a British Standard-approved sharps bin, which is destroyed by incineration or other approved method (see part (a) of figure). The inappropriate disposal of sharps presents a risk, not only to doctors and nurses, but also to staff such as laundry workers and domestic assistants. In addition, laundry workers have to handle heavily blood-contaminated and tissue-contaminated sheets and clothes, increasing their risk of acquiring infections such as hepatitis B (see parts (b) and (c) of figure). These groups of workers should be offered vaccination against hepatitis B infection.

(g) HIV and tuberculosis

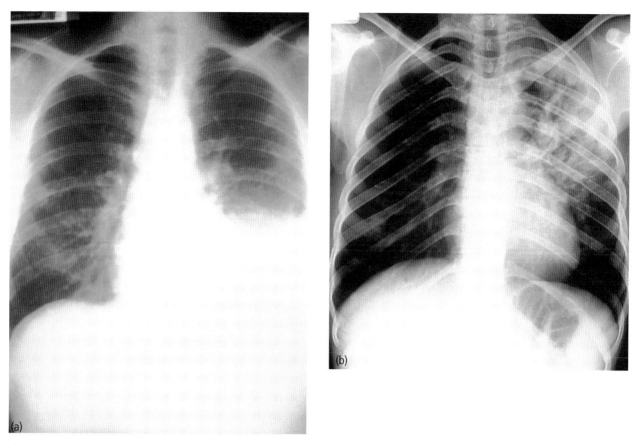

Figure 16.9 Manifestations of TB in HIV-positive patients: (a) pleural effusion; (b) cavitation. (a) Copyright S.C. Stenton. Reproduced with permission. (b) Copyright Edmund Ong. Reproduced with permission.

There is conflicting epidemiological evidence concerning whether healthcare workers are at increased risk of contracting tuberculosis compared to the general population. However, a recent study has suggested that this remains the case. HIV infection in either staff or patients is another risk factor for tuberculosis. Multi-drug-resistant infection of healthcare workers has been described. Such cases have been associated with high mortality and rapid disease progression. Procedures in hospitals such as sputum induction and aerosol treatments increase the risk of exposure to infected respiratory secretions. Consequently, there is a significant possibility of healthcare workers coming into contact with sputum-positive patients before the diagnosis has been made. Mortuary workers are another occupational group considered to be at an increased risk of tuberculosis. The protection of workers against infection comprises the assessment of medical history and hypersensitivity to purified protein derivative (PPD), appropriate offers of bacille Calmette–Guérin (BCG) vaccination and adherence to safe working practices.

(h) Leptospirosis

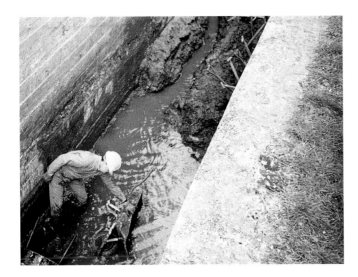

Figure 16.10 Risk of exposure to leptospirosis during canal clearance. Copyright Christine J. Meusz. Reproduced with permission.

The presence of water assists the acquisition of a number of zoonotic infections. Leptospirosis is caused by pathogenic serovars of *Leptospira interrogans*. *Leptospira icterohaemorrhagiae* causes Weil's disease; its principal reservoir is the rat. Leptospirosis is an occupationally acquired infection in those circumstances in which workers are likely to come into contact with infected rat urine or an infected animal. In the UK, the occupational groups at risk include farmers, dairy workers, sewer and canal workers. Globally, people working in rice fields, on sugar or banana plantations or in mines may be at risk. The incidence of leptospirosis is seasonal, with the peak incidence during the summer months in the UK. The clinical presentation is usually of fever, headache, muscle pains, photophobia and jaundice, rarely progressing to renal failure in severe cases of infection. Treatment is with antibiotics but severe infections may require intensive support in hospital.

(i) Malaria

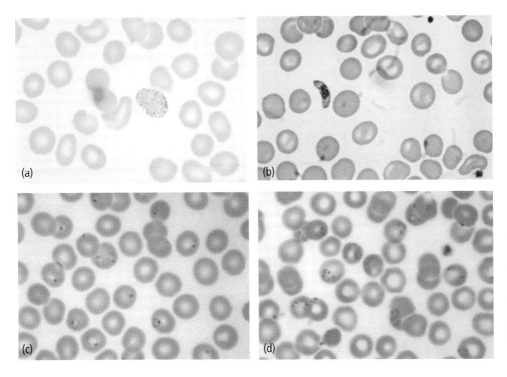

Figure 16.11 Haematological appearances of malaria infection: (a) amoeboid stage of *Plasmodium vivax*; (b) male gametocyte in *Plasmodium falciparum* infection; (c) heavy parasitization with *Plasmodium falciparum*, with evidence of multiple parasites in some cells; and (d) *Plasmodium falciparum*. Copyright M.H. Snow. Reproduced with permission.

Malaria remains an important infectious disease to consider whenever travel to Africa, Asia or Latin America is being proposed. The illness may be caused by four species of *Plasmodium*: *falciparum*, *vivax*, *ovale* and *malariae*. Approximately

2000 infected individuals enter the UK each year, more than half of whom are infected with *Plasmodium falciparum*. Infection begins when the female anopheline mosquito inoculates sporozoites into the body. The sporozoites are taken up into the liver very rapidly. Merozoites then enter the bloodstream, where they invade red blood cells. Inside red blood cells the merozoites either divide asexually to produce more merozoites or differentiate to produce gametocytes. The latter may subsequently be ingested by other mosquitoes to complete the life cycle.

A diagnosis of malaria can be made by examining blood films. It is usual to request a thick and a thin film. The appearance depends on the type of malaria. In falciparum malaria, the most serious infection, there are lots of small ring forms, double nuclei, appliqué-form and crescent-shaped gametocytes. Enlarged red blood cells with eosinophilic Schüffner's dots characterize *P. vivax*, and oval fringed cells with Schüffner's dots are associated with *P. ovale*. It is important to have a high index of suspicion of malaria in anyone with an unexplained fever who has been in an endemic area. Treatment will depend on the species of *Plasmodium* and the sensitivity to drugs. Guidelines for the prevention of malaria in travellers abroad are available from travel centres and are reviewed regularly and updated.

(j) Methicillin-resistant *Staphylococcus aureus*

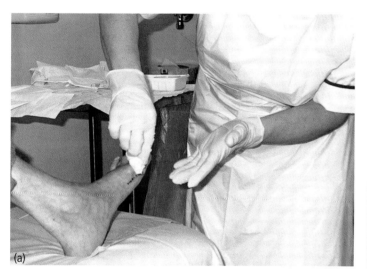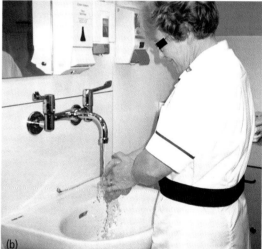

Figure 16.12 Methicillin-resistant *Staphylococcus aureus* infection: (a) elderly patient with wound; (b) effective hand washing as a control measure to reduce spread of MRSA. Copyright Nerys R. Williams. Reproduced with permission.

Healthcare workers may present a risk to immunocompromised patients as methicillin-resistant *Staphylococcus aureus* (MRSA) can be colonized in the nose, throat, axillae and perineum of the worker. The organism can also become established in damaged skin and on the hands of those with active eczema and dermatitis. The condition can be very difficult to treat in healthcare workers and may be fatal in patients undergoing chemotherapy or those who are immunocompromised by neoplastic and other diseases. The spread of MRSA within a hospital can lead to the closure of surgical theatres as attempts are made to eradicate it. Healthcare workers colonized by MRSA that has proved resistant to eradication and whose jobs are such that the risk to patients is significant, e.g. in intensive care units, may need permanent redeployment. Even non-colonized healthcare workers can spread the infection, hence the need for scrupulous hand washing and changing of barrier garments such as gloves and aprons.

(k) Mites

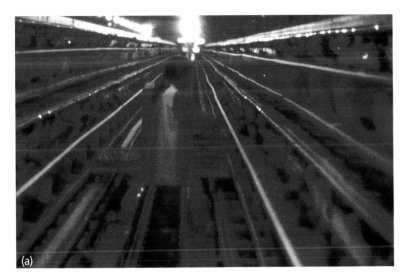

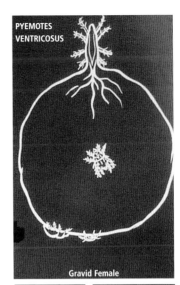

Figure 16.13 Mite infestation in poultry farming: (a) battery hens; (b) life cycle of pyemotes. Copyright Margaret Anne Harrison. Reproduced with permission.

Rashes at work may occur due to infestations and many occupational groups may be affected, from nurses to seamen. Poultry workers may also become infested with mites, as they tend birds that are kept in confined spaces. *Pyemotes ventricosus* is the mite that has been implicated in outbreaks amongst such workers. It lives on the grain used to feed the birds and sometimes transfers to humans, preferring warm and moist parts of the body.

(l) Mycobacteria

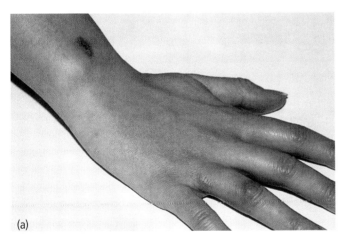

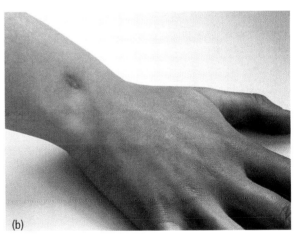

Figure 16.14 *Mycobacterium marinum* infection in pet shop worker: (a) acute, (b) healing. Copyright M.H. Snow. Reproduced with permission.

Mycobacteria may be classified into obligate parasites (*Mycobacterium leprae*, *M. tuberculosis* and *M. bovis*), environmental saprophytes and occasional parasites, the long list of which includes *M. avium*, *M. intracellulare*, *M. marinum* and *M. ulcerans* and non-pathogenic saprophytes. *M. avium* and *M. intracellulare* infections have become prominent because of their association with HIV infection. *M. marinum* causes cutaneous and soft tissue infections. It can be acquired by humans from the sea and rivers or from fish tanks and aquariums. The organism needs a temperature less than 37°C to grow. Characteristically, mild abrasions of the skin lead to the formation of a granulomatous lesion that often heals spontaneously. However, if deeper tissues become infected, it may be necessary to treat with either anti-tuberculous drugs or other antibiotics, such as trimethoprim or minocycline. Because of the widespread occurrence of *M. marinum* amongst marine life, infections of fishermen, fishmongers or pet shop workers, as in the case shown, are occasional occupational diseases.

(m) Myiasis

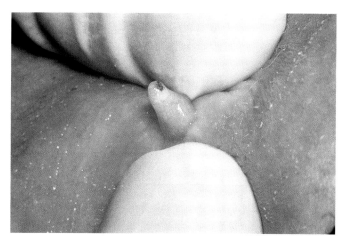

Figure 16.15 Maggot removed from soldier on exercise in Belize. Copyright M.H. Snow. Reproduced with permission.

Most business trips to foreign countries do not involve much risk of exposure to many of the indigenous infections because visitors rarely venture beyond the confines of a modern hotel. However, when it is necessary to go into the field, there is the possibility of exposure to a wide range of infections, some of which may be difficult to prevent. Vaccinations help to protect workers from well-known infections, such as typhoid, hepatitis A, yellow fever etc. However, workers will remain vulnerable to bites from insects and from contact with water, which can carry a variety of infective organisms. The slide shows a maggot from the Tumba fly being removed from a soldier. Myiasis is the infestation of an organ or tissue by dipterous larvae. However, human myiasis is relatively uncommon. Usual sites for the deposition of maggots are orifices, wounds or open epithelial surfaces of sleeping people. Symptoms vary according to the site of entry and the type of fly concerned. Some infestations are benign and asymptomatic. Others, for example the screw worm larvae, are directly invasive and cause pain and discomfort. Removal of the larvae may be difficult and this is sometimes done under local anaesthetic by surgical extraction. Direct application of turpentine or ether to the tissue may assist the extraction.

(n) Orf

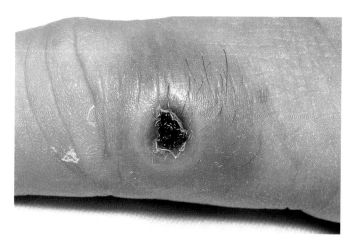

Figure 16.16 Cutaneous orf in a sheep farmer. Copyright M.H. Snow. Reproduced with permission.

Orf is also known as contagious pustular dermatitis and is caused by a pox virus. Occupational groups at risk of this condition, which is acquired from sheep, include farmers, abattoir workers, vets and butchers. The condition presents in the early stages as a dark-red papule, usually on the fingers or, more rarely, the lips. The lesion enlarges until it reaches 1–4 cm in diameter, becomes umbilicated and develops a softened centre containing clear fluid and pus. There may be local tenderness and systemic upset. Complete recovery without scarring takes place within 3 weeks.

(o) Typhus

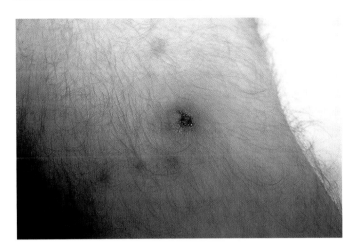

Figure 16.17 Eschar of scrub typhus. Copyright M.H. Snow. Reproduced with permission.

Outdoor workers may be at risk of acquiring rickettsial diseases following bites from ticks, mites or fleas. The main infections are Rocky Mountain spotted fever, epidemic, murine and scrub typhus and Q fever. The rash illustrated occurred in a tennis coach in Zimbabwe. Murine typhus, or endemic typhus, occurs worldwide. The organism *Rickettsia mooseri* is transmitted by fleas from the reservoir in rodents. There is a flu-like illness culminating in rigors, severe frontal headache and fever that lasts for about 10 days. The rash begins in the axillae or on the arms. It then becomes generalized, with a macular or maculopapular appearance. Unlike Rocky Mountain spotted fever or epidemic typhus, it does not become haemorrhagic. This type of typhus is not usually fatal in previously healthy people. Tetracycline antibiotics are specific treatments for rickettsial infections. In countries with poor sanitation and hygiene, people working in granaries or food stores are at risk of this infection.

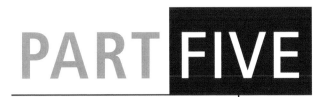

PART FIVE

WORK AND MENTAL HEALTH

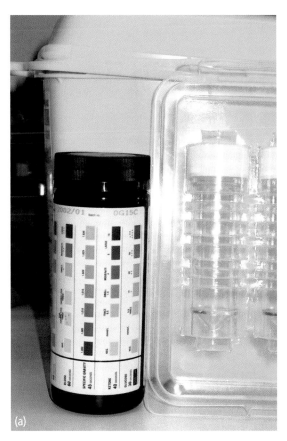 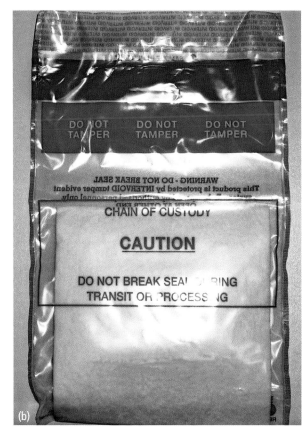

Figure 17.1 Screening for substance abuse. (a) Urine test: anti-tampering procedure. (b) Chain of custody: tamper-proof bag. Copyright John Harrison. Reproduced with permission.

Routine drug testing is common in the USA but relatively uncommon in the UK. Some industries, such as offshore, conduct routine pre-employment drug screening and many workplaces are increasingly looking at both pre-employment and random testing. Individuals working in safety-critical posts such as train driving are subject to testing post-accident. Companies planning on introducing testing programmes for existing employees need to ensure that the procedures carried out are rigorous and that they have systems for dealing with positive results. Some illegal substances are eliminated from the body quickly (e.g. heroin), whereas others can take weeks for complete clearance (e.g. cannabis).

There are ethical issues to be considered before implementing a drug-screening programme. Guidance is available in the UK from the Faculty of Occupational Medicine. Important aspects of any programme are ensuring that specimens obtained do come from the individual being tested and the establishment of a chain of custody when sending the specimens to the laboratory for analysis. The sample provided should have its temperature and specific gravity checked. In the presence of the individual being tested, the sample is divided into two parts, which are placed in plastic tubes. The tubes are sealed and the donor signs them. They are placed in a transport package and sent to the laboratory. There should be a system for checking the identity of the donor when the package reaches the laboratory and a system for safeguarding the communication of the results of testing. If the sample in one of the tubes is positive, the other is tested. A combination of measurement techniques is used to maximize sensitivity (detecting positives) in the first sample and specificity (detecting negatives) in the second sample.

18 Shift work and extended hours of work

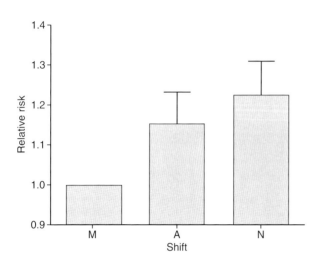

Figure 18.1 Shift work and accidents: the relative risk of industrial injuries on the morning (M), afternoon (A) and night (N) shifts. Redrawn with permission from material prepared by Simon Folkard based upon original data in L. Smith, S. Folkard, & C.J.M. Poole, Increased injuries on night shift. *Lancet* 1994; **344**:1137–9.

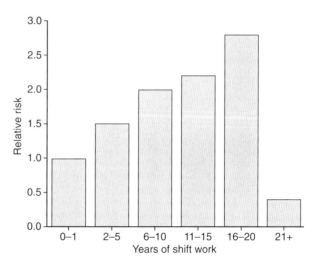

Figure 18.2 Heart disease and shift work: the relative risk of ischaemic heart disease in shift workers (relative to day workers) as a function of years of experience of shift work. Redrawn with permission from material prepared by Simon Folkard based upon original data in A. Knutsson, T. Akerstedt, B.G. Jonsson, & K. Orth-Gomer, Increased risk of ischaemic heart disease in shift workers. *Lancet* 1986; **2**:89–92.

A complete assessment of the workplace should include an enquiry into patterns of work. Many types of work require employees to work unsocial hours, e.g. manufacturing processes operating for 24 hours per day or service industries. There are many different types of shift patterns, but the modern trend is for workers to be employed on continental shifts: working 12-hour rotating shifts. There is some evidence that working shifts can have adverse effects on health and lead to an increased incidence of accidents. There appears to be an increased prevalence of angina, hypertension and morbidity due to ischaemic heart disease and an increased risk of myocardial infarction in shift workers. The first graph demonstrates a higher relative risk of accidents occurring during an afternoon or night shift, compared to the risk during the morning shift. The *a priori* level of risk throughout the 24-hour period was considered to be constant, correcting for possible confounding factors. The second graph shows an increasing relative risk of ischaemic heart disease with years of shift work, compared to day workers.

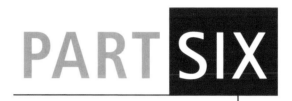

PART SIX

OCCUPATIONAL LUNG DISORDERS

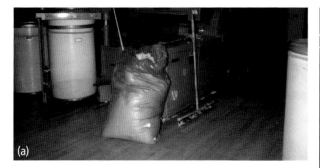

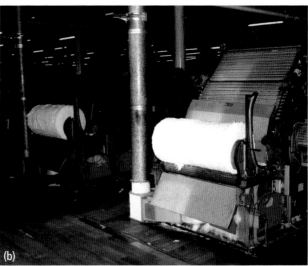

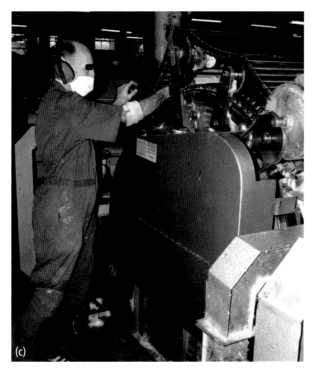

Figure 19.2 (a), (b) and (c) Cotton making: carding. Copyright Angela Fletcher. Reproduced with permission.

Byssinosis was clinically graded by Roach and Schilling in 1960. More recently, a World Health Organization (WHO) classification has been produced. There is consensus that symptoms progress from occurring occasionally, on Mondays, to occurring on other days, with evidence of permanent respiratory disability due to reduced ventilatory capacity. The latter is quantified in the WHO classification. However, prospective studies of the progression of the disease in individuals are lacking. The prevalence of byssinosis depends on the quality and airborne concentration of the cotton dust to which workers are exposed. The highest prevalences have been described in opening room operatives (where bales of cotton are opened after delivery) and card room workers (carding is a type of combing procedure that prepares the cotton for spinning). Byssinosis is least prevalent amongst ring spinners (ring spinning is a later stage of the process of cotton spinning).

Reference

S.A. Roach, and R.S.F. Schilling, A clinical and environmental study of byssinosis in the Lancashire cotton industry. *British Journal of Industrial Medicine*, 1960; **17**: 1–9.

20 Occupational asthma

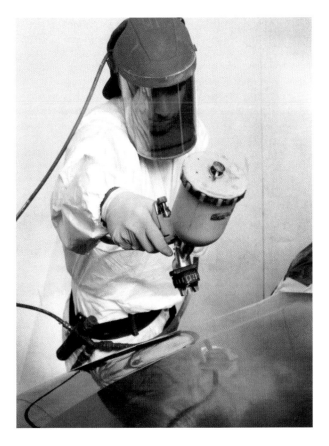

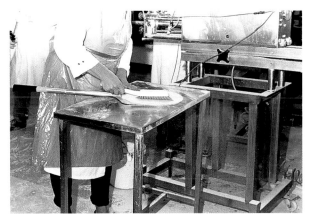

Figure 20.2 Exposure to flour dust. Reproduced with permission from the Health & Safety Laboratory, Sheffield, UK.

Figure 20.1 Isocyanate paint spraying, one of the commonest causes of occupational asthma in the UK. Courtesy of the Health & Safety Executive, UK. Crown copyright material is reproduced with the permission of the Controller of Her Majesty's Stationery Office.

Exposure to flour dust is common in bakeries and is associated with dermatitis and occupational asthma. The exact agent in the flour that causes sensitization is the subject of much debate. Flour dust itself as well as added improvers and amylase have all been suggested. Prevention involves the control of flour dust and the implementation of respiratory and skin health surveillance programmes. The diagnosis of occupational asthma involves history, clinical examination, 2-hourly peak flow measurements and assay of specific IgEs. This will be informed by knowledge of the workplace hazards and the likelihood of inhalation of the putative agent.

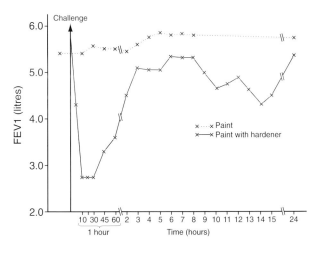

Figure 20.3 Results of bronchial challenge test. Redrawn with permission from original supplied by C.A.C. Pickering.

In some cases measurements of respiratory function and/or immunological testing provide evidence to support the diagnosis. In some cases, however, it becomes necessary to consider challenging the affected worker with the substance that is thought to be the cause of the asthma. This is most likely to be required when the substance is not a known asthmogen, when there are several possible causes of asthma and the worker's future employment depends on knowing the cause, when the severity of asthma is such that further workplace exposures should be avoided and when the diagnosis remains in doubt after other investigations have been completed. The aim is to conduct a single-blind exposure in controlled conditions. Measurements of airway responses include forced expiratory volume in 1 second (FEV1) and forced vital capacity (FVC) or peak expiratory flow (PEF), before and after the challenge. Testing should continue for at least 24 hours afterwards. Tests of non-specific airway responsiveness, such as a methacholine challenge, may be carried out where the concentration of methacholine required to produce a 20 per cent decrease in FEV1 (PC20) is measured. This can be done to obtain a baseline measurement and following a return to the workplace after a period away from work.

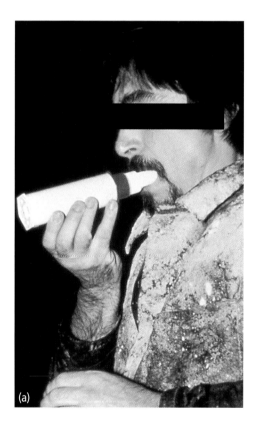

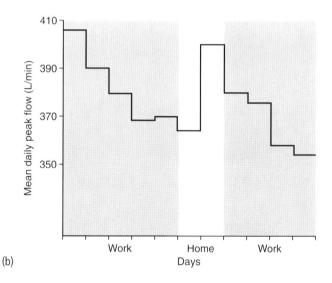

Figure 20.4 (a) Worker using a mini peak flow meter. (b) Chart of results, suggesting occupational asthma. Copyright P.S. Burge. Reproduced with permission. (b) Redrawn with permission from original supplied by C.A.C. Pickering.

Serial measurements of PEF rates can provide useful supporting evidence when occupational asthma is suspected. A mini peak flow meter may be carried easily, facilitating the performance of frequent measurements, both at work and at home. The worker must be instructed how to use the meter correctly, typically taking the best of three readings. Ideally he or she should make recordings every 2 hours during the whole day over a period of several weeks. It is also helpful if the recording period includes a holiday or period away from work that is more than 2 days. Readings are recorded in a diary and the worker is asked to record whether there have been any symptoms during the day, treatment taken, if any, and any particular work activities. The results are often expressed as maximum, minimum and mean PEF rates for each day. A pattern of gradual reduction in flow rates during the time at work followed by an increase when away from work suggests occupational asthma. However, other patterns may occur.

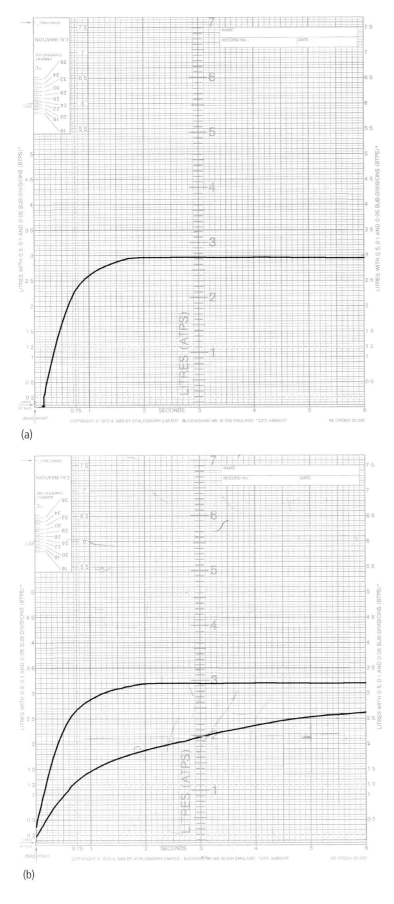

(a)

(b)

Figure 20.5 Pitfalls of spirometry: (a) origin missing; (b) failure to achieve at least two consistent traces indicating maximal effort. Copyright John Harrison. Reproduced with permission.

Simple spirometry is an invaluable tool in occupational medicine for the initial assessment of respiratory problems and for conducting health surveillance of workers exposed to respiratory hazards. The dry wedge spirometer is popular because it is easy and cheap to use and calibrate and it gives reproducible results,

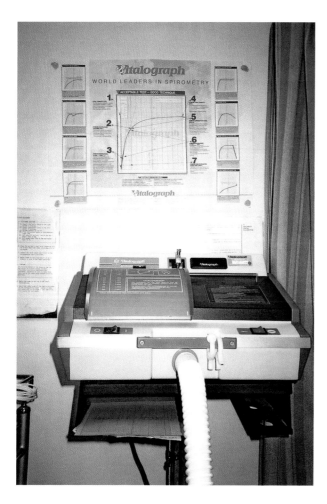

Figure 20.6 Spirometry equipment. Copyright John Harrison. Reproduced with permission.

as long as the correct technique is used. Operators require instruction about how to use the equipment, and the subject being assessed must be schooled and then observed whilst performing the investigation. A certain amount of encouragement is required to obtain the best results. Effort is required from the subject, and a sub-optimal result is unacceptable. The stylus must be positioned correctly on the chart before beginning. The subject must continue to exhale, following a full inhalation, for a minimum of 6 seconds. In cases of airflow obstruction, a 12-second machine may be required to ensure that a full expiration has been achieved. FEV1, FVC and the FEV1:FVC ratio are the results that are used most often.

Chapter 21 | Extrinsic allergic alveolitis

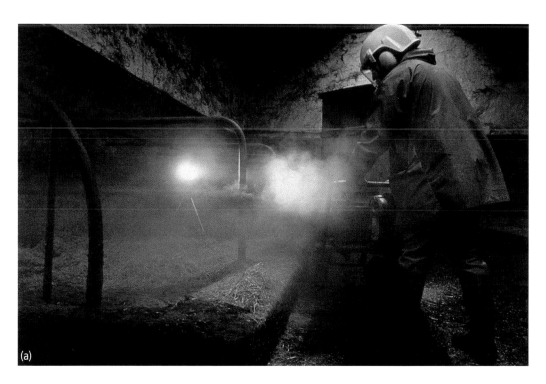

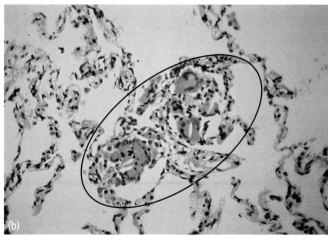

Figure 21.1 (a) Mushroom cultivation. Copyright Margaret Anne Harrison. Reproduced with permission. (b) Granuloma in a section of lung. Copyright Anthony Newman-Taylor. Reproduced with permission.

Mushrooms are grown commercially on compost. The indoor environment is warm and very humid, typically 60°C and 100 per cent humidity. Mushroom spawn is added to the compost and a large number of spores may be generated. Inhalation of these organic spores can lead to the development of extrinsic allergic alveolitis, a granulomatous inflammatory reaction caused by an immunological response to the spores. The disease is called mushroom worker's lung when it occurs in this occupational setting. The many other examples of extrinsic allergic alveolitis include farmer's lung, malt worker's lung and bagassosis.

Chapter | 22 Diseases due to inorganic dusts

(a) Asbestosis

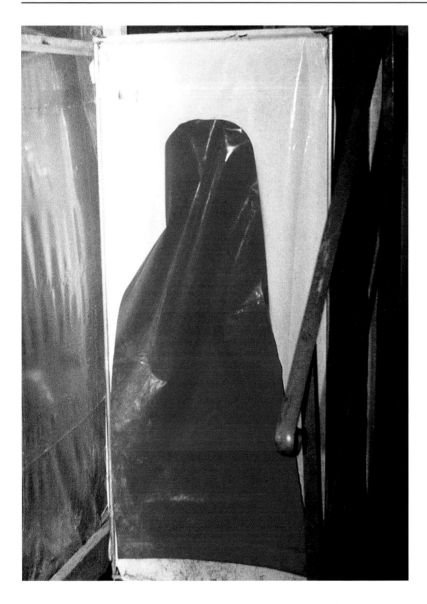

Figure 22.1 Asbestos stripping/hazard control. Copyright John Harrison. Reproduced with permission.

Possibly one of the main sources of asbestos exposure now is its removal from buildings. Public concern about the dangers of being exposed to asbestos has led to pressures to have it removed whenever it is found. Asbestos sheeting that is in good condition only poses a risk to building occupants when building work takes place and unless this happens it should be left undisturbed. When it becomes necessary to remove asbestos, the area must be sealed off to avoid the dispersal of asbestos fibres. A tent is used to facilitate entry and exit from the sealed area, to ensure fibres are not carried on clothing or allowed to escape through broken seals.

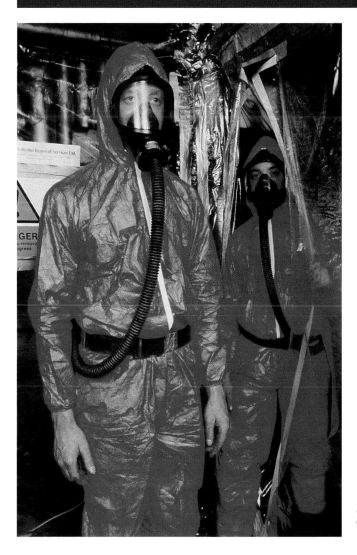

Figure 22.2 Workers wearing personal protective equipment for asbestos stripping. Courtesy of the Health & Safety Executive, UK. Crown copyright material is reproduced with the permission of the Controller of Her Majesty's Stationery Office.

Personal protective equipment (PPE) is one way to protect workers from workplace hazards. However, it should be used only when other methods of reducing exposure to hazards have been explored. Asbestos stripping is an example of a job that requires wearing not only a full body suit, but also an air-fed respirator. Work is carried out in an enclosed space and workers may suffer from heat stress. In the UK, there is a statutory requirement for biennial medical examinations of designated asbestos workers that include auscultation of the chest and spirometry.

See also 'Worker protection' (page 113).

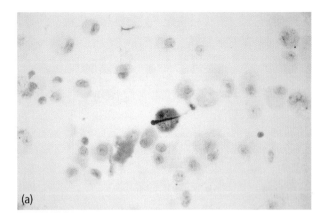

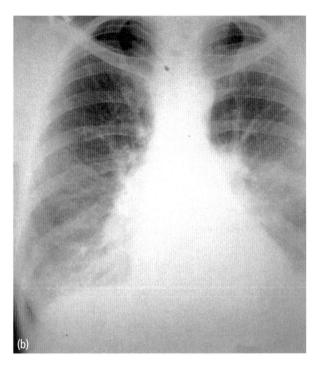

Figure 22.3 Asbestosis: (a) asbestos body; (b) chest x-ray showing lower zone fibrosis (asbestosis). Copyright C.A.C. Pickering. Reproduced with permission.

Asbestosis is a pulmonary fibrosis resulting from the inhalation of asbestos, which is a fibrous silicate. Exposure to high levels of asbestos fibres has been associated with the development of bilateral opacities in the lower zones of lung fields on chest x-rays. Typically, there is irregular linear shadowing that becomes honeycombed in appearance as the disease progresses. Clinically, end-expiratory crackles can be heard on auscultation of the chest and there may be finger clubbing. Because the radiological appearance of asbestosis is not pathognomonic of the condition, other pointers towards the diagnosis should be sought. The existence of pleural plaques may be helpful. Similarly, the finding of an asbestos body (fibres coated with a protein–ferritin complex) in the sputum supports a history of previous asbestos exposure.

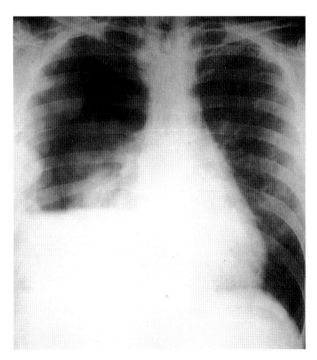

Figure 22.4 Chest x-ray showing pleural effusion. Copyright C.A.C. Pickering. Reproduced with permission.

In addition to lung fibrosis and bronchial carcinoma, diseases of the pleura may occur in workers exposed to asbestos fibres. Pleural effusions may be either benign or malignant. They may be bloodstained, recurrent and bilateral. The occurrence of blood in the fluid raises the possibility of a mesothelioma, and benign pleural effusions may progress to this, although it is rare. Effusions may be associated with pleural thickening, which may or may not progress to limit chest expansion on one or both sides of the chest. Bilateral diffuse pleural thickening is associated with exposure to high levels of asbestos and it may restrict ventilation of the lower part of the lung. A high-resolution computed tomography (CT) scan of the chest is required to distinguish this pleural disease from underlying parenchymal fibrosis. Extensive bilateral diffuse fibrosis is a prescribed disease.

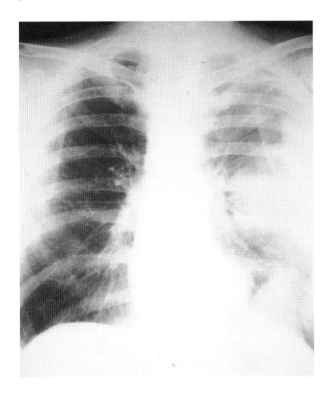

Figure 22.5 Chest x-ray of mesothelioma. Copyright C.A.C. Pickering. Reproduced with permission.

A mesothelioma is a tumour arising from the mesothelium of one of the body's serous cavities, usually the parietal pleura. In most developed countries, asbestos is the most frequent cause of mesothelioma. This invariably lethal tumour is also a prescribed disease. The diagnosis is often difficult because of the variable histological patterns that may be seen in biopsy specimens. The opinion of several pathologists may be required in some cases. Needle biopsies and even open biopsies may be unreliable. Immunochemical staining techniques may assist the diagnosis. The tumour increases in size within the pleural cavity, although it may erode outwards. A pleural effusion is present in about two-thirds of the cases. This may lead to marked shift of the mediastinum (which may be the cause of the symptoms) on presentation. Drainage of the effusion will reveal the tumour on x-ray as an irregular opacity arising from the parietal pleura, but CT scans can be very helpful, even in the presence of fluid.

(b) Coal worker's pneumoconiosis

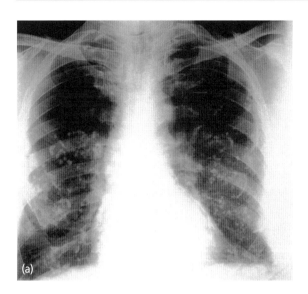

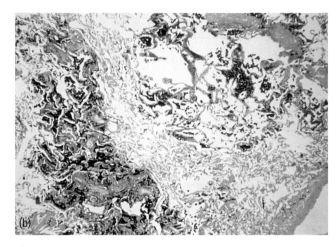

Figure 22.6 Effects of chronic exposure to coal dust: (a) radiological 'emphysema' and (b) carbon accumulation in lungs and emphysematous changes. Copyright C.A.C. Pickering. Reproduced with permission.

This condition develops after relatively high cumulative exposures to underground coal mine dust, usually over a period of more than 20 years. The features of simple coal worker's pneumoconiosis result from the accumulation of dust in the lung parenchyma and the tissue reaction that ensues. Typical chest radiographic appearances are lung fields containing scattered small, rounded opacities. The removal of men from exposure at this stage usually prevents the progression to complicated pneumoconiosis and the development of respiratory impairment. In cases where respiratory impairment does occur, there is usually an obstructive pattern of lung function loss, the chest radiograph reveals irregular opacities in the lung fields and there are pathological changes of emphysema and fibrosis surrounding centrilobular collections of dust-laden cells. Although the situation has been somewhat confused because of the need to allow for the effects of cigarette smoking, there is now good evidence of the occurrence of emphysema in non-cigarette smoking coal workers with a history of heavy dust exposure.

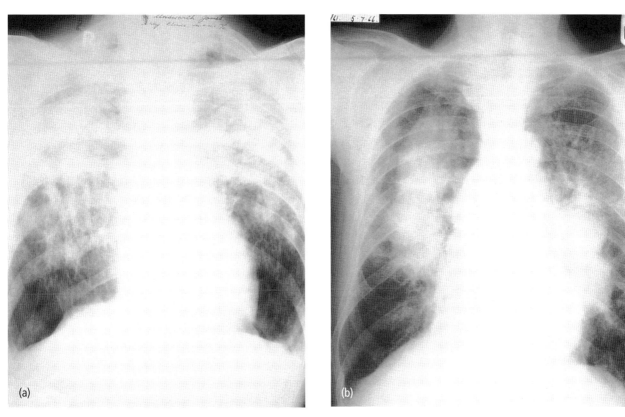

Figure 22.7 Chest x-rays showing extensive progressive massive fibrosis. Copyright C.A.C. Pickering. Reproduced with permission.

Progressive massive fibrosis (PMF) is an example of complicated coal worker's pneumoconiosis, with characteristic x-ray changes and the occurrence of disabling symptoms. PMF is said to exist when one or more x-ray nodules is more than 1 cm in diameter. A typical chest x-ray appearance is that of a mass in the upper or middle zone, oval in shape and with the long axis parallel to the pleura. It has a smooth outline. Eventually the mass may cavitate and lead to the production of copious amounts of black material (melanoptysis). The cavity may become infected, forming a mycetoma. The lung function loss is mainly obstructive, resulting from the space-occupying effects of the masses and scar emphysema occurring on a background of heavy simple pneumoconiosis and emphysema.

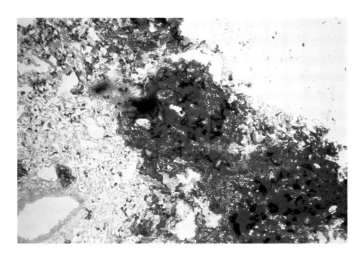

Figure 22.8 Carbon deposition in the lungs. Copyright C.A.C. Pickering. Reproduced with permission.

The deposition of carbon in the lungs has been considered to be harmless, although there is some evidence from research into the effects of exposure to diesel exhaust that heavy deposits in the lungs may overwhelm the scavenging protective mechanisms and lead to inflammatory changes. Whether this is due to chemicals adsorbed onto carbon particles remains to be determined conclusively.

See also 'Silicosis – slate worker's pneumoconiosis' (page 91).

(c) Silicosis

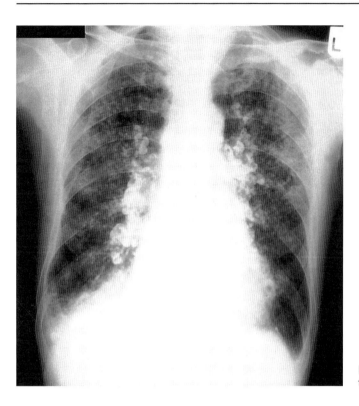

Figure 22.9 Chest x-ray showing silicosis and eggshell calcification in the hilar regions. Copyright C.A.C. Pickering. Reproduced with permission.

Silicosis results from the inhalation of one of the three crystalline forms of silicon dioxide. The most common of these is quartz, heavy exposures to which cause acute silicosis. It causes alveolar damage leading to the accumulation of protein-rich fluid and inflammatory cells. This is then followed by lung fibrosis, which causes a restrictive respiratory defect on spirometry, reduced gas transfer and hypoxaemia. This form of silicosis may be rapidly fatal. Chronic (active) silicosis frequently resulted from industrial exposures to respirable quartz before improvements in occupational hygiene in developed industrial countries. The disease is still a major problem in developing countries. Lesions appear on chest x-rays before the development of symptoms. Shadows in the upper zones, or evenly distributed throughout the lung fields, are rounded opacities. They are often associated with enlargement of lymph nodes in the hilar region. In the absence of continuing exposure to silica, the nodules may become inactive and they calcify from the periphery inwards. When this occurs in hilar lymph nodes, the x-ray appearance is called 'eggshell calcification'.

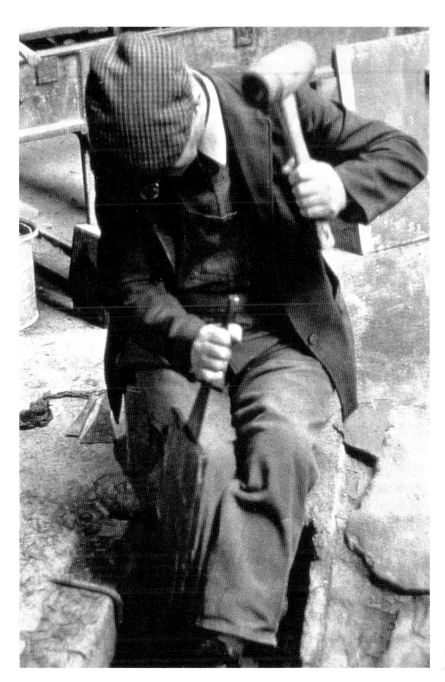

Figure 22.10 Slate cutter. Copyright Margaret Anne Harrison. Reproduced with permission.

In the UK, slate is obtained from mines and quarries in North Wales. Because it shatters easily, it has to be cut by hand. Slate contains 15–35 per cent crystalline quartz (sometimes higher from other sources). Consequently, slate cutters may be exposed to silica each time they break a piece of slate. A puff of dust is released when the sheets of slate separate. Slate worker's pneumoconiosis has been recognized for more than a century. The jobs with most exposure were 'getting' the slate underground and 'dressing' of roof slates indoors. Silicosis resulting from slate cutting has been reported to be characterized by a large amount of bilateral hilar gland enlargement and eggshell calcification, even in the absence of radiological evidence of lung fibrosis. Wet working methods and dust extraction should be employed in slate cutting to make it safe from the risk of pneumoconiosis.

Chapter 23

Problems associated with indoor air in non-industrial workplaces

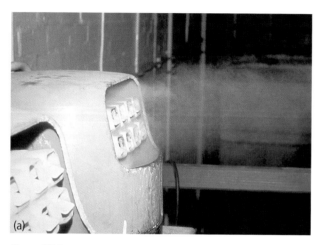 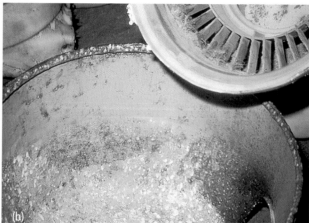

Figure 23.1 Spinning disc humidifier: (a) exterior; (b) interior showing accumulated deposits. Copyright C.A.C. Pickering. Reproduced with permission.

Humidification of indoor air may be achieved by various means. The illustration shows a spinning disc humidifier using cold water to produce water droplets that are circulated into the air. Contamination of water in cold-water humidifiers has been associated with the occurrence of humidifier fever. The symptoms are similar to those of extrinsic allergic alveolitis and include fever, myalgia, headache, breathlessness and wheezing. Typically, attacks occur on the first day back at work after a weekend or a holiday. Spirometry may reveal a restrictive picture and there may be a decrease in transfer factor. However, the chest x-ray is always normal. Research into the cause of humidifier fever does not support a single organism being responsible. Whether it results from an immunological response to microorganisms or from the production of endotoxin remains to be determined.

PART SEVEN

OCCUPATIONAL DISEASES OF THE SKIN

Chapter 24 Occupational diseases of the skin

(a) Contact dermatitis

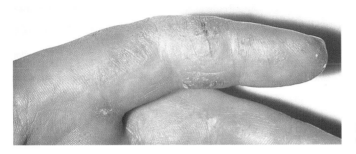

Figure 24.1 Chronic dermatitis. Copyright Janet McClelland. Reproduced with permission.

Dermatitis, or eczema, is a very common occupational disease. Contact irritant dermatitis occurs when the skin is damaged by contact with irritant substances. A previous history of atopic eczema is a risk factor for this type of dermatitis. Allergic contact dermatitis is less common than contact irritant dermatitis, but its occurrence may lead to sufferers having to change jobs because of the difficulty in protecting them from further exposures. Skin damaged by heat or degreasing is a risk factor for this type of dermatitis. A sub-acute onset of contact irritant dermatitis is characterized by redness, scaling and fissuring of the skin. Painful fissures (keens) on the knuckles, nail folds and palms are seen in chronic dermatitis.

(i) Irritant

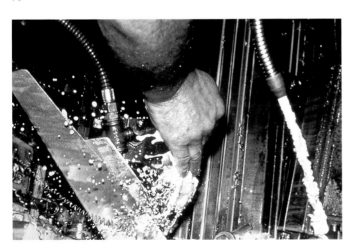

Figure 24.2 Exposure to metal-working fluids. Courtesy of the Health & Safety Executive, UK. Crown copyright material is reproduced with the permission of the Controller of Her Majesty's Stationery Office.

Contact dermatitis is not uncommon in the engineering industry. One well-known cause is an oil–water mixture often called 'white water'. This is used during machining, e.g. with a lathe. It acts as a lubricant and a coolant. In fact it is usually a cocktail of chemicals including antibacterial compounds, such as isothiazolones, and detergents. Operators often do not wear gloves to protect their skin, claiming that they interfere with machine operation. The risk of developing contact irritant dermatitis is increased if the concentration of the white water increases, or if the sump is not cleaned out frequently.

(ii) Allergic

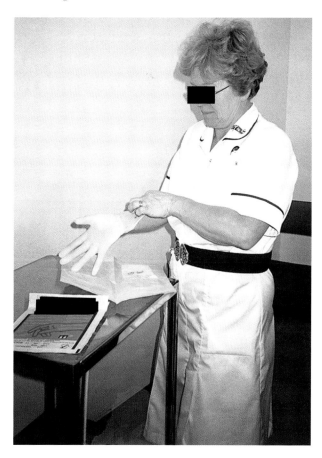

Figure 24.3 Latex allergy: asthma due to latex may result from the inhalation of dusting powders as latex gloves are put on or removed. Copyright Nerys R. Williams. Reproduced with permission.

Latex is one of the more recently recognized causes of occupational asthma and dermatitis. The increasing incidence of these conditions has been attributed to the increased use of rubber gloves by healthcare workers as a response to the greater awareness of the risks of acquiring the human immunodeficiency virus (HIV), and associated acquired immune deficiency syndrome (AIDS), and hepatitis B infections. Latex is derived from the sap of the *Hevea brasiliensis* tree, which provides the raw material for gloves, condoms, balloons and catheters. The majority of cases are thought to be due to the inhalation of latex from the dusting powders present in the gloves as a means to assist the wearer in putting them on. Risk groups include nurses, laboratory technicians and, more recently, garage workers who are protecting their hands against used engine oils. An individual sensitized to latex may have urticaria, rhinitis or conjunctivitis, or occupational asthma. Skin prick tests are available to assist with the diagnosis, as is the radioallergosorbent test (RAST), which measures IgE levels in the blood. The prevalence of latex allergy has been estimated to be up to 17 per cent in laboratory technicians and up to 14 per cent in nurses and physicians.

Once sensitized, there are wider implications for individuals, as latex is found in the home and cross-reactions can occur with fruits such as avocado and banana. Anaphylactic reactions have been described and can be so severe that individuals are unable to work, for example on wards where others are using latex gloves. Prevention is through the use of low-latex or non-latex gloves. The sensitized individual needs counselling about sources of latex within other healthcare environments, e.g. dentistry, and at home and may also be advised to wear an allergy identification tag. If the person has suffered from anaphylaxis, an additional precaution is the carriage of an emergency adrenaline (epinephrine)-containing kit.

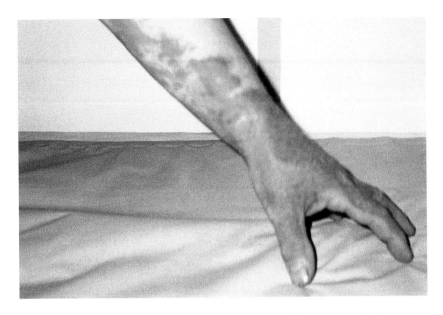

Figure 24.4 Epoxy dermatitis. Copyright Nerys R. Williams. Reproduced with permission.

Epoxy resins are widely used in adhesives because of their strong binding properties. They also occur in specialized paints and together with their curing agents, which may be plasticizers, solvents or diluents, can act as severe sensitizers should they come into contact with the skin. They become much less dangerous when cured. Epoxy resins may also be used as binders for glass-fibre filling material and when dermatitis occurs in relation to the handling of glass fibre, the involvement of any epoxy resins also needs to be evaluated.

(b) Photodermatitis including phytophotodermatitis

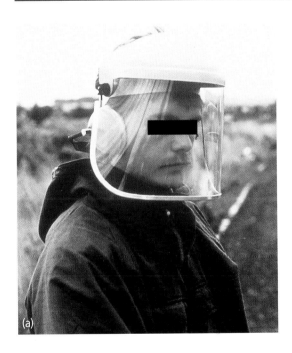

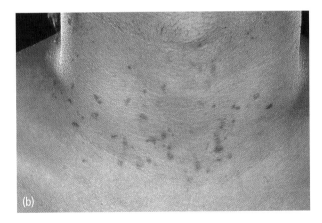

Figure 24.5 A strimmer operator: (a) protective clothing; (b) photodermatitis on the neck. Copyright Margaret Anne Harrison. Reproduced with permission.

The man in picture (a) works outdoors, cutting grass at the side of the road. He uses a strimmer. The rash on his neck is an example of a phytophotodermatitis (illustration b). Many plants and lichens cause this and in the UK the Compositae are the commonest cause. Other plants include the giant Russian hogweed and the pea family. Strimmers macerate the vegetation, scattering a mixture of solid and liquid material that will come into contact with exposed skin unless it is protected. Ultraviolet light from the sun interacts with a naturally occurring psoralen (furocoumarin) to produce the dermatitis. In-vitro tests have shown the psoralens to be mutagenic.

Strimmers are also noisy and they expose the operator to hand–arm vibration. See also 'Vibration (hand–arm and whole body)' (page 28).

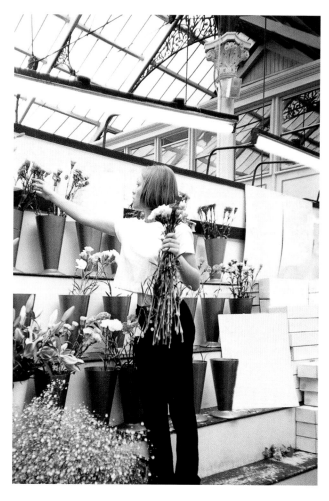

Figure 24.6 Florist at flower stall. Copyright Nerys R. Williams. Reproduced with permission.

A typical florist's shop contains a variety of workplace hazards. Irritant dermatitis may arise from contact with certain types of plants, as well as from wet working and handling metal wire. Handling the bulbs of plants such as daffodils may also cause a problem. Primulae, chrysanthemums, tulips and daffodils may cause sensitization. In addition, photodermatitis may occur (phytophoto-dermatitis) following contact with certain plants (see above) and exposure to ultraviolet light in sunlight. Contact urticaria may also occur when in contact with certain cacti.

(c) Other conditions: non-malignant

(i) Oil folliculitis

This rash is due to a folliculitis of the hair-bearing skin of the backs of the hands, arms, thighs, abdomen, face and neck. Hair follicles become blocked by come-dones, leading to the development of inflammatory papules and pustules. It is caused by exposure to petroleum oils, such as those used in metalworking. Mineral and other oils are included in the European schedule of occupational diseases, which is a list of occupational diseases drawn up by the European Commission for member states to consider for inclusion into national legislation to permit the payment of compensation. In the UK, non-infective dermatitis of external origin is already a compensatable condition.

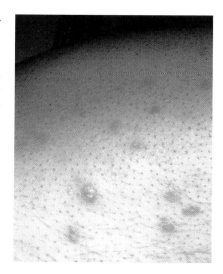

Figure 24.7 Oil folliculitis. Reproduced from *Hunter's Diseases of Occupations*, edited by P.J. Baxter, P.H. Adams, T.C. Aw, A. Cockcroft and J.M. Harrington, published in 2000 by Arnold with permission of R.J.G. Rycroft.

(ii) Chloracne

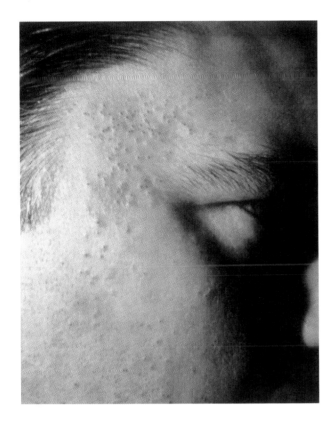

Figure 24.8 Chloracne. Reproduced from *Hunter's Diseases of Occupations*, edited by P.J. Baxter, P.H. Adams, T.C. Aw, A. Cockcroft and J.M. Harrington, published in 2000 by Arnold with permission of R.J.G. Rycroft.

This specific skin condition occurs when certain poly-halogenated chemicals come into contact with the skin. The term chloracne is perhaps a misnomer, as it suggests that is only chlorinated chemicals that exert this effect. Typical lesions of chloracne are distributed over the temples, behind the ears and on the male genitals. The rash may spread to involve the trunk and limbs. The lesions are comedones and pale-yellow cysts. Inflammation may be seen in severe cases. Chloracne is said to be a marker of systemic absorption of the relevant chemical.

Perhaps the best publicized chemicals causing chloracne are in the dioxin family, such as the 2,3,7,8-tetrachlorodibenzo-p-dioxin (TCDD) released in the Seveso incident in Italy in 1976, which is an intermediate used in the manufacture of 2,4,5-trichlorophenol. Other industrial accidents have exposed workers to dioxin. The clinical effects in exposed workers include chloracne, peripheral neuropathy, hepatic damage, hypercholesterolaemia and hepatic porphyria.

(d) Cancers

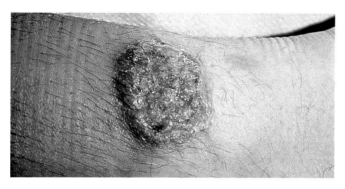

Figure 24.9 Carcinoma of the skin on the arm. (a) Copyright Margaret Anne Harrison. Reproduced with permission.

Skin cancer in the form of carcinoma of the scrotum in chimney sweeps is a historical example of cancer developing in an occupational group exposed to a specific hazard. Squamous cell carcinoma is associated with exposure to polycyclic aromatic hydrocarbons, which are found in soot, tar, pitch and bitumen. Unrefined mineral oils are also carcinogenic and they may cause carcinoma of the skin if there is prolonged contact. The risk is increased if there is concomitant exposure to ultraviolet light, particularly in people with fair skin.

See also 'Occupational cancers' (page 105).

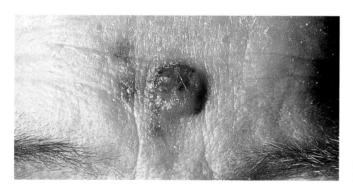

Figure 24.10 Malignant melanoma on the forehead. Copyright Janet McClelland. Reproduced with permission.

The incidence of malignant melanoma is increasing. There is epidemiological evidence of its association with exposure to sunlight in some countries, such as Australia. The rates of incidence are higher amongst non-manual professional people, suggesting that intermittent exposure, rather than continual exposure, may be important. This idea has been supported in a study of navy personnel, which showed that those working indoors had higher rates compared to those working both indoors and outdoors. The finding of high rates of melanoma in airline pilots has suggested that a combination of in-flight ultraviolet radiation exposure and travel to hot countries may be important.

Basal cell carcinoma of skin has a characteristic appearance and location. It begins as a slow-growing, flattened nodule of the skin of the face, usually in a restricted area in front of the ears, above the mouth and below the supra-orbital ridges. Later, the centre breaks down to form a shallow ulcer. The periphery of the nodule persists to form a smooth, slightly raised margin, which develops into a characteristic rolled edge. Early diagnosis is important to secure successful treatment of this condition. Awareness of possible occupational causes such as exposure to polycyclic aromatic hydrocarbons and ultraviolet light will help to promote a low threshold of suspicion for the possibility of this type of cancer. Sunlight is an important cause, and the avoidance of sunburn during outdoor work is prudent. It is also associated with chronic exposure to arsenic, as are squamous cell carcinoma and Bowen's disease (intraepithelial carcinoma *in situ*).

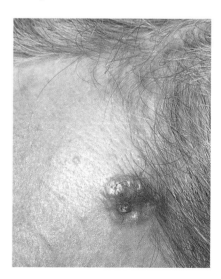

Figure 24.11 Basal cell carcinoma (rodent ulcer). Copyright Janet McClelland. Reproduced with permission.

(e) Investigations

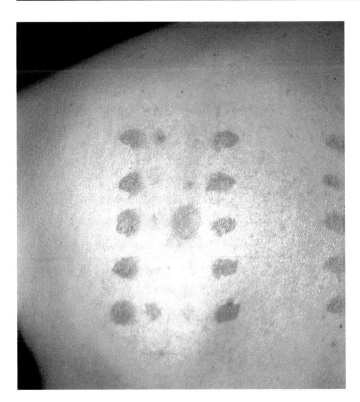

Figure 24.12 Patch testing using the skin of the back. Copyright Janet McClelland. Reproduced with permission.

The purpose of patch testing is to detect contact allergy. The preferred site for testing is the back. A standard battery of commercially available tests is often used. The suspected substance is applied to the skin in a standardized manner and the patches are left in place for 48 hours. The tests are read at 48 and 96 hours to see if an eczematous reaction has occurred at the site of the patch. There are many pitfalls in carrying out patch testing, and so it is advisable to perform it in specialist clinics. The risks of patch testing include an eruption on the patient's back or a flare-up of existing eczema. There is also a possibility of causing sensitization. False-positive and false-negative reactions may occur if substances are irritants or if the concentration being tested or the vehicle is wrong.

25 Occupational cancers

(a) Liver cancer

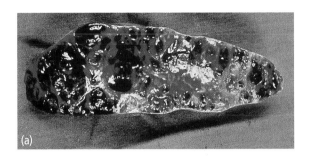

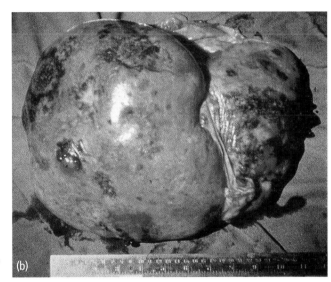

Figure 25.1 (a) and (b) Adenocarcinoma of the liver. Copyright Anthony Yardley-Jones. Reproduced with permission.

Hepatocellular carcinoma is a liver cancer of global importance. Hepatitis B and hepatitis C viral infections are risk factors for its development, as is the ingestion of aflatoxins. Other occupational exposures that may increase the risk are polychlorinated biphenyls (PCBs) and trichloroethylene. There are over 200 possible isomers of PCBs, which are manufactured by the chlorination of biphenyl. PCBs are used as heat insulators in heavy-duty electrical transformers and capacitors. They are difficult to destroy, and persist in the environment once released. There is animal evidence of their carcinogenicity and limited evidence that they are human carcinogens. Trichloroethylene is considered to be a probable carcinogen (Group 2A) by the International Agency for Cancer Research (IARC). Epidemiological studies have demonstrated an increased risk for liver and biliary tract tumours, as well as for non Hodgkin's lymphomas.

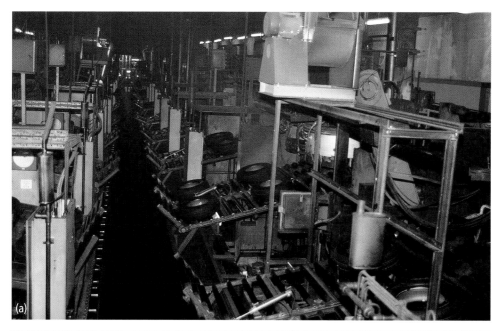

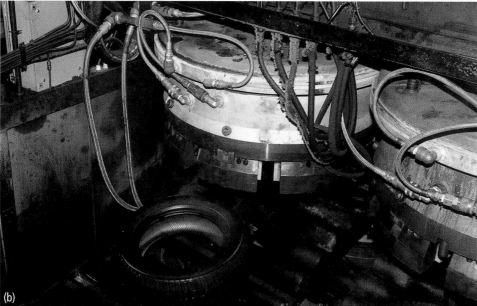

Figure 25.2   (a) and (b) Causes of cancer: the later stages of rubber tyre manufacture. Copyright Alastair Leckie. Reproduced with permission.

The rubber used to make pneumatic tyres is a complex mixture of chemicals, including accelerators, antioxidants and solvents. It was for this reason that earlier editions of *Hunter's Diseases of Occupations* stated that it was inadequate to ascertain that a man is *just* a rubber worker, for at least three harmful substances may be handled in the rubber trade. Hunter referred to benzene, carbon disulphide and lead monoxide. It later became clear that the chemical β-naphthylamine, an established bladder carcinogen in the dyestuffs industry, was also present in the rubber mixing process. Its use is now prohibited. However, α-naphthylamine is not considered to be a bladder carcinogen, tumours occurring when this chemical has been used being attributed to contamination with β-naphthylamine. This demonstrates the importance of the position of a chemical side-chain in determining carcinogenicity.

(b) Bladder cancer

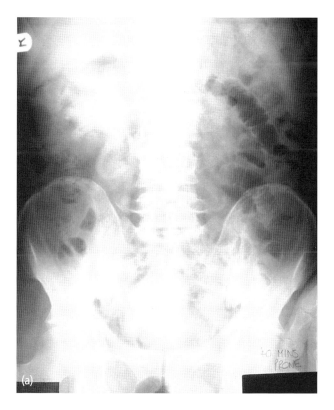

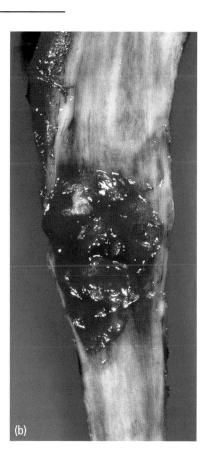

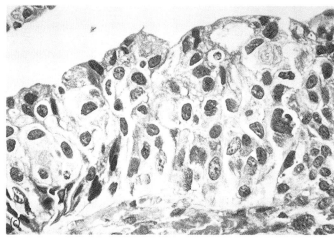

Figure 25.3 Clinical slides illustrating bladder cancer: (a) Intravenous urogram filling defect; (b) pathology; (c) histology. Copyright David Neal. Reproduced with permission.

Bladder cancer is the eighth most common cancer in men. The majority are transitional cell tumours and present in the seventh decade. Tobacco consumption is an associated lifestyle risk factor in Western countries. Bladder cancer due to occupation presents 10–15 years earlier than in the general population. The industries that have been directly implicated in causing exposures to bladder carcinogens are the rubber, gas and dyestuffs industries. Historically, the first cases were recorded by Rehn in 1895, when three cases of bladder tumours were found amongst 45 men preparing fuchsine. It was shown later that the incidence of this tumour was 33 times greater amongst dye workers than in the general male population. Aromatic amine benzidine-based dyes have been shown to be specific bladder carcinogens.

(c) Leukaemia

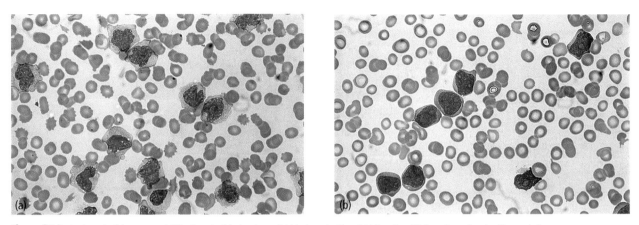

Figure 25.4 Leukaemia: (a) acute myeloid leukaemia; (b) chronic myeloid leukaemia. Copyright Jonathan Wallace. Reproduced with permission.

There are many different types of leukaemia and a well-known association between the development of leukaemia and exposure to ionizing radiation. Following a brief exposure, there is an increased risk of developing acute lymphoblastic or acute myeloid leukaemia initially. Chronic myeloid leukaemia may develop at a late stage. However, the incidence of chronic lymphocytic leukaemia is not increased. It has been estimated that the dose to double the natural incidence of leukaemia lies between 0.3 and 0.5 Gy. Apart from ionizing radiation, there is a well-established relationship between exposure to benzene and the occurrence of acute myeloid leukaemia. An increased risk of leukaemia has been reported in electrical workers, print workers and workers in the rubber industry. However, the causative agent(s) is unknown. It has been suggested also that electromagnetic radiation may be implicated in causing leukaemia, particularly in children. However, recent studies have not confirmed a causal link between exposure to electromagnetic radiation and cancer in humans.

See also 'Ionizing radiations' (page 42).

(d) Lymphoma

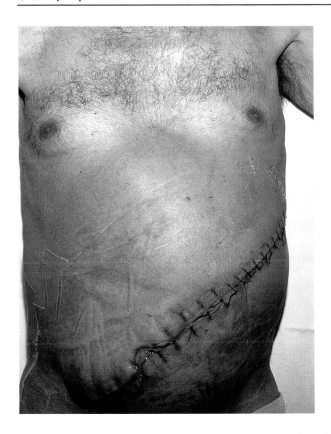

Figure 25.5 Splenectomy in a patient with a lymphoma. Copyright John Harrison. Reproduced with permission.

The main indications for splenectomy are trauma, hereditary spherocytosis, chronic idiopathic thrombocytopaenic purpura and staging laparotomy for Hodgkin's disease and non-Hodgkin's lymphoma. Industrial processes causally associated with the occurrence of lymphoma have been found in the rubber industry. Ionizing radiation is associated with non-Hodgkin's lymphoma, and this type of lymphoma has been shown to have a higher incidence in individuals previously diagnosed as having skin cancer. It has been suggested that immunosuppression by ultraviolet light might be an explanation for this. Phenoxy acid herbicides and some chlorinated organic compounds (trichloroethylene, tetrachloroethylene and PCBs) have also been implicated as causes of non-Hodgkin's lymphoma.

See also 'Ionizing radiations' (page 42) and 'Skin cancer' (page 102).

Reference

D. Hunter, *The Diseases of Occupations*. The English Universities Press Ltd, London, 1957.

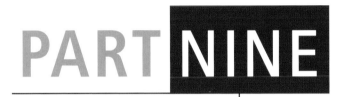

PART NINE

WORKER PROTECTION AND WORKPLACE ASSESSMENT

26 Worker protection

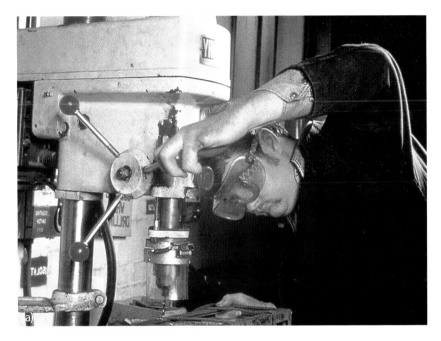

Figure 26.1 Drill operation. Copyright Margaret Anne Harrison. Reproduced with permission.

Operating a drill may be a hazardous procedure. Foreign bodies may enter the eye, causing penetrating injuries and possible loss of eyesight. Another possibility is that the drill bit may become unattached and fly off, causing severe injury; the bit should be protected by a guard. Drills such as these are often poorly designed from an ergonomic perspective. The operator has to adopt an awkward posture to use the drill, which may have to be sustained for some time. Pre-existing problems with the neck or upper limbs would affect an operator's ability to use such equipment.

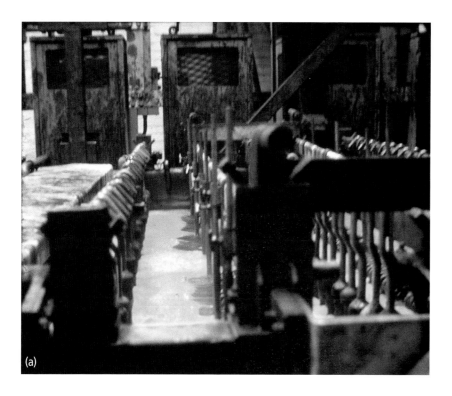

(a)

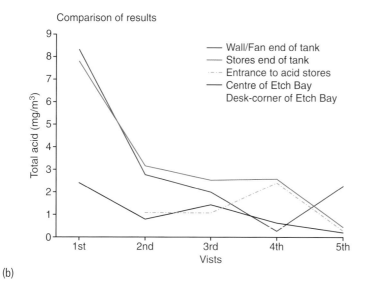

Comparison of results

— Wall/Fan end of tank
— Stores end of tank
--- Entrance to acid stores
— Centre of Etch Bay
Desk-corner of Etch Bay

(b)

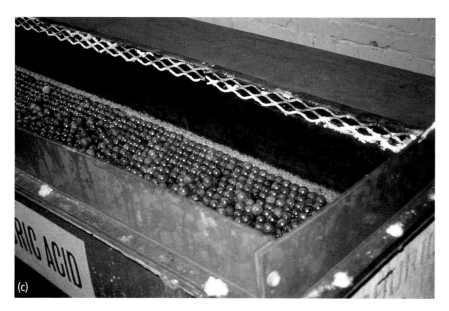

(c)

Figure 26.2 Hazard control: (a) a sulphuric acid etching tank; (b) graph of acid in air measurements versus introduction of control measures; (c) the same tank with plastic spheres. Copyright David Foster and Gordon Smith. Reproduced with permission.

The Control of Substances Hazardous to Health Regulations require employers to minimize risks to health by controlling exposures to workplace hazards. The reduction of concentrations of substances in air may be achieved by a number of methods. For example, measurements of sulphuric acid in air were taken at set distances away from an open tank in the work setting shown in the illustration. On each occasion, a new control method was introduced. At the first visit, the only control was a roof-sited fan. At the second visit, plastic spheres were placed on the surface of the acid. At the third visit, lip ventilation had been introduced, with a flange along one side of the tank. For the fourth visit, a new, more powerful fan had been added to the lip ventilation; and at the fifth visit, a new substance was in the tank which was an equal mixture of sulphuric and nitric acids plus oxidizing agents and inorganic salts. No plastic spheres were used at the time of the fifth visit. Although ventilation is an important method of controlling emissions it can be seen that, in the workplace being studied, the largest decreases in airborne concentration were effected by covering the tank with plastic spheres or by substituting the sulphuric acid with an alternative substance. This study also highlights the important role of the occupational hygienist in controlling workplace exposures.

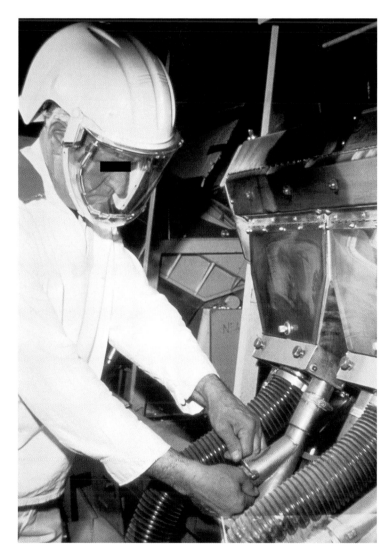

Figure 26.3 Use of an air-fed helmet. Copyright C.A.C. Pickering. Reproduced with permission.

The diagnosis of occupational asthma can have serious implications for workers. The management of occupational asthma aims for early diagnosis, identification of the cause or causes and the avoidance of further exposure. The last factor may often mean relocation, redeployment or loss of employment. Once an individual has become sensitized to an asthmagen, asthmatic responses may be triggered by further exposures to very low concentrations of it. The use of respiratory protection, such as an air-fed helmet, may allow workers to continue in their current job, at least in the short term. However, in the long term, complete avoidance of further exposure to the cause must be sought. The use of helmets is not an alternative to eliminating or minimizing exposures to respiratory sensitizers.

See 'Occupational asthma' (page 77).

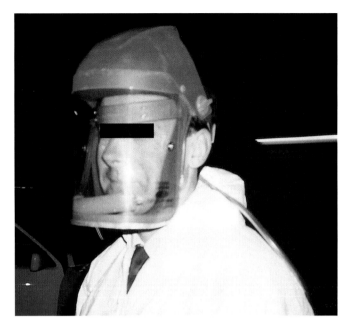

Figure 26.4 Full face air-fed mask used in spraying of isocyanates in motor vehicle repair. Copyright Nerys R. Williams. Reproduced with permission.

The photographs show the standard personal protective equipment worn by workers spraying isocyanate-containing paints. The mask is fed by a supply of air via a line. The air flows over the face, producing a clean air breathing supply, and then passes out. Complications can arise if there is contamination of the air supply with oils, either from air compressors or from the intake zone. The masks are usually on personal issue and are re-usable. Workers also wear disposable paper overalls to protect the skin and clothing.

See also 'Occupational asthma – paint spraying' (page 77).

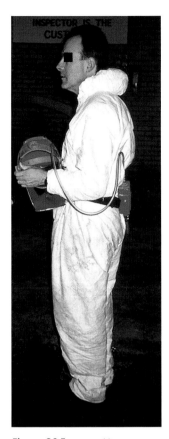

Figure 26.5 Disposable paper overalls worn during spraying of paints. Copyright Nerys R. Williams. Reproduced with permission.

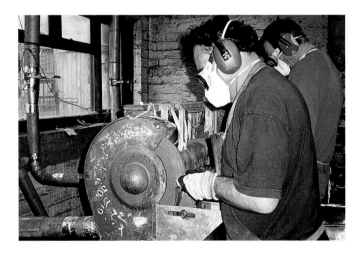

Figure 26.6 Man polishing brass wearing ear defenders and mask. Copyright Nerys R. Williams. Reproduced with permission.

The polishing of brass involves potential exposure to lead, hand–arm vibration and noise. To protect against noise, the worker is wearing ear defenders – cup-like muffs that cover the whole ear. In hot conditions, the rubber seals that lie in direct contact with the ear can become sweaty and so sweat-absorbent disposable stick-on pads are available. Deterioration of the rubber seals leads to reduced function of the muffs. Workers who are claustrophobic may object to using muffs, but a range of hearing protection equipment is available, including plugs. Cotton wool will not protect the ears from noise and should never be used.

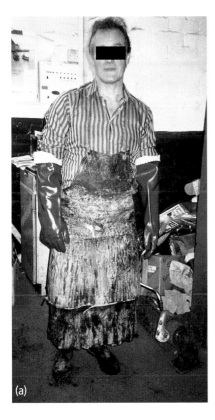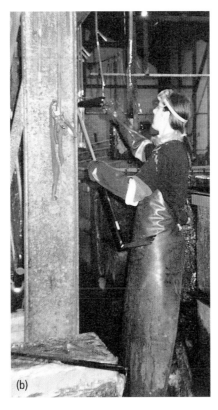

Figure 26.7 (a) and (b) Personal protective equipment worn during chromium plating. Copyright Nerys R. Williams. Reproduced with permission.

Chromic acid is corrosive. When items are being plated and workers need to lift them in and out of baths of acid, they need to ensure that their skin does not become contaminated, as this may lead to ulcers, burns or dermatitis. The illustration shows a plater wearing gauntlets, apron and wellington boots. The extent of contamination during the process can be seen by the amount of chrome on the apron and boots of the plater in (a). Other equipment usually worn includes a visor or goggles to protect the eyes against splashes, as seen in (b). (Note that in this case goggles are not being worn over the eyes!)

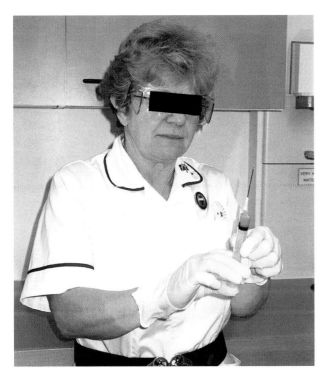

Figure 26.8 Eye and skin protection for the drawing up of injections. Copyright Nerys R. Williams. Reproduced with permission.

Several medical procedures, such as joint injections, require the preparation of mixtures of local anaesthetic and steroid. There is a risk of accidental exposure from splashes to the eyes or contamination of the skin, both when drawing up solutions and when the joint is injected.

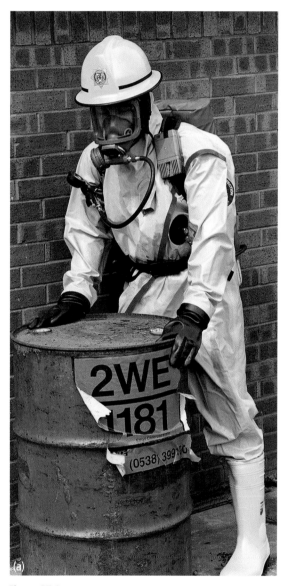 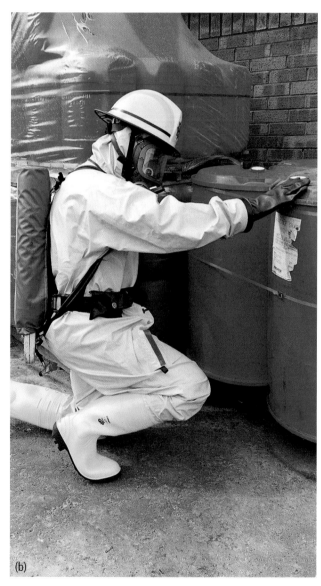

Figure 27.1   (a) and (b) Fire officers inspecting a chemical drum. Copyright Chris Ide. Reproduced with permission.

Fire fighters often have to deal with potential or actual exposures to chemicals when they attend a fire or an accident. Their training includes the careful evaluation of such situations and the use of chemical suits and breathing apparatus. They must be physically fit to wear this type of protective equipment, which is relatively heavy, cumbersome and hot to wear. Information about chemicals can be obtained from the computer databases used by the fire and rescue services, e.g. CHEM-DATA, or from the manufacturer, in the form of HAZTEXT cards if the chemicals are being transported, or material safety data sheets (MSDS). The labelling of chemicals is a statutory requirement under labelling regulations.

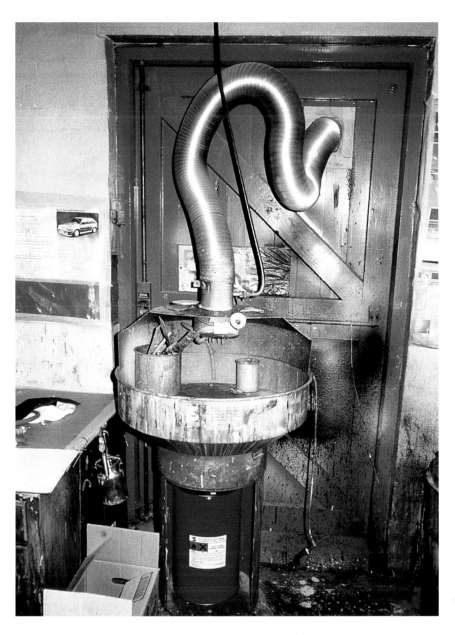

Figure 27.2 Local exhaust ventilation for solvent mix. Copyright Nerys R. Williams. Reproduced with permission.

Exposure to solvent fumes can produce symptoms of headaches, light headedness, nausea and reduced consciousness. The control of such exposure involves the use of local exhaust equipment, which draws the fumes away from the breathing zone of the worker. Many systems are custom built, but this illustration is an example of a home-made exhaust system designed to remove fumes given off during a paint-mixing process. Such equipment needs to be regularly checked to ensure that the airflow is sufficient to remove fumes. This can be done with a specific instrument or, more crudely, with a smoke tube for daily checks.

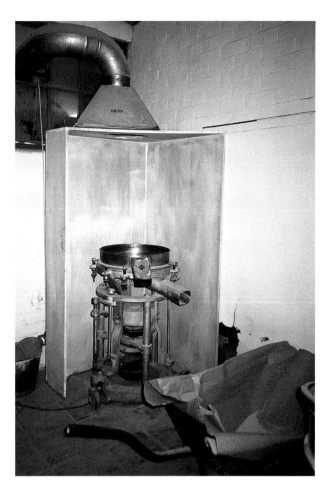

Figure 27.3 Hazard control: local exhaust ventilation around an enclosed mixer. Copyright Nerys R. Williams. Reproduced with permission.

Effective ventilation reduces the concentration of inhaled substances in the workplace. Where natural ventilation provides insufficient air exchanges, mechanical devices are used. Mechanical ventilation may be employed to supply an area with outside air or to extract air to the outside. In some circumstances, ducting is chosen, as the air may be moved considerable distances. The performance of ventilation systems must be checked regularly. This may involve measuring air volume flow rates, velocities and air pressures at extraction points or inside ducts. These measurements must be performed by suitably trained professionals, such as occupational hygienists.

Many types of activity may generate aerosols. Substances that are inhaled in the workplace include gases, vapours, fumes, mists, dusts and fibres. Activities such as bagging, debagging, transferring between containers, agitating, stirring, spraying, sanding and planing may liberate airborne aerosols. For many substances, occupational exposure standards exist, and the role of ventilation systems is to ensure that airborne concentrations do not exceed the set limits, as part of an overall strategy to control risks to health.

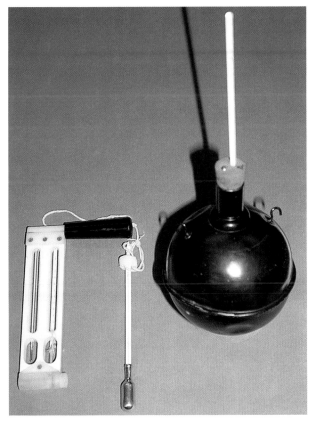

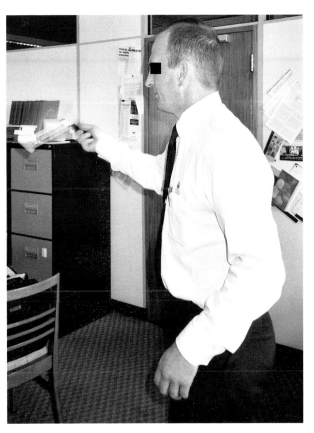

Figure 27.4 Occupational hygiene instruments for measuring thermal climate: whirling hygrometer, Kata thermometer and globe thermometer. Copyright John Harrison. Reproduced with permission.

Figure 27.5 Use of a whirling hygrometer to assess environmental conditions in an office. Copyright Nerys R. Williams. Reproduced with permission.

Some occupations expose workers to extremes of temperature. The heat balance of the body depends on the rate of gain versus the rate of loss of heat. The amount of heat stored in the body is the amount of heat generated by metabolism plus the net heat gain or loss resulting from radiant heat exchange, convective heat exchange, conductive heat exchange and evaporative heat loss. Measurements of heat stress require measurements of these factors, or surrogate measurements of them. The whirling, or sling, hygrometer is a simple yet reliable method of measuring the dry bulb air temperature and the wet bulb temperature of the air. The percentage relative humidity or water vapour pressure may be obtained using a psychrometric chart. The globe temperature gives an indirect assessment of radiant temperature and the Kata thermometer gives an estimate of air velocity. Indices of heat stress may be computed using different combinations of these measurements, such as the effective temperature, corrected effective temperature and the wet bulb globe temperature (WBGT) index.

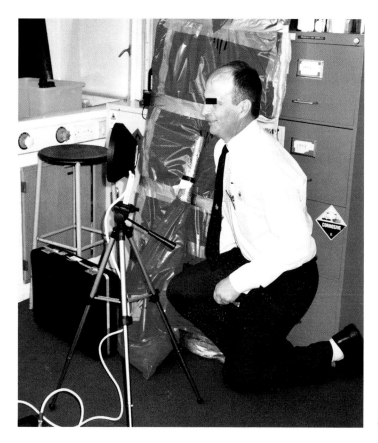

Figure 27.6 Use of a lamp to show the Tindall beam effect. Copyright Nerys R. Williams. Reproduced with permission.

Used to identify dust, aerosols and liquid colloids, the Tindall lamp in this illustration shines light and can be used to identify leaks from gaskets on ducts on local exhaust ventilation systems.

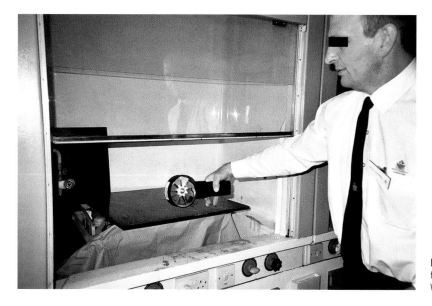

Figure 27.7 Use of a rotary anemometer to measure face velocity of a fume cupboard. Copyright Nerys R. Williams. Reproduced with permission.

When the rotating vane in the illustration reaches a steady speed, the air velocity can be read in metres per second. With the model shown, the size of the duct can be entered and the volume flow rate will be calculated automatically. This device is useful because it operates over a wider surface than the smaller hot wire anemometer, so is less prone to vortex effects. However, it is battery operated, and therefore not considered to be intrinsically safe, and cannot be used in flammable atmospheres.

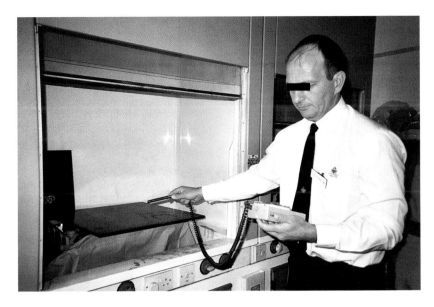

Figure 27.8 Use of a hot wire anemometer. Copyright Nerys R. Williams. Reproduced with permission.

Also known as an electro-thermal anemometer, the hot wire anemometer consists of a thermistor which is held in a hole drilled into the end of the probe. As the air travels across the thermistor, it cools the wire and the resistance increases. This increase is measured in the machine and displayed as metres per second or feet per minute. Much smaller than the rotating vane anemometer, the hot wire can be placed inside ducting to measure airflow. A series of readings is needed rather than a single reading because of the small area over which flow is measured. Like the rotating anemometer, the hot wire device cannot be used in flammable atmospheres because it is not intrinsically safe.

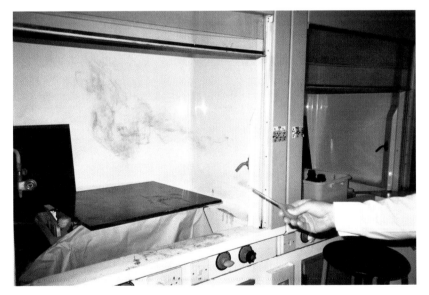

Figure 27.9 Use of a smoke tube to test airflow at a fume cupboard. Copyright Nerys R. Williams. Reproduced with permission.

A smoke tube is selected to trace air movement rather than to measure airflow. The results demonstrate the capture efficiency of local exhaust ventilation and can be used to test for leaks in asbestos enclosures. The equipment is easy to use and cheap to buy. It can also be employed to look at general airflow within a factory environment, but care must be taken not to direct the smoke at an individual, as it contains crystals coated in sulphuric acid which are an irritant to the eyes or if inhaled.

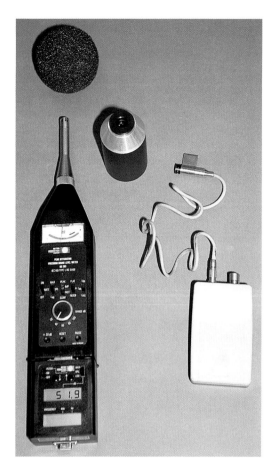

Figure 27.10 Occupational hygiene equipment for measuring noise. Copyright John Harrison. Reproduced with permission.

Noise is measured using a noise level meter. Personal noise exposures are assessed by dosimetry (the device on the right of the illustration). The machines in many workplaces are often noisy and it is not unusual for levels of noise to exceed those associated with damage to hearing. In such circumstances employers must provide their workers with information about the effects of noise, and hearing-protection devices should be made available to be worn if requested.

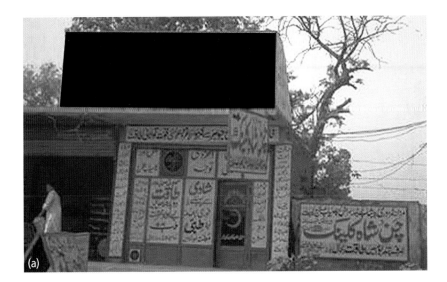

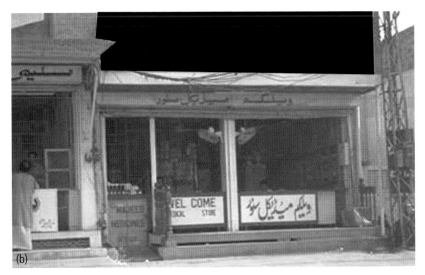

Figure 27.11 (a) and (b) Working overseas: local medical facilities in rural India. Copyright G.M. Helliwell. Reproduced with permission.

A major concern for companies operating internationally is to ensure the health, safety and welfare of their employees when they travel abroad. Workers must travel on behalf of their companies to seek new markets, assist with the installation of new plant and with the maintenance of existing plant, or merely for meetings. Such workers may become ill as a result of gastrointestinal illness, infection, accidents, physical assault or because of the occurrence of a constitutional illness. Consequently, there is an expectation that corporate occupational physicians will familiarize themselves with the local healthcare facilities in the relevant countries. Outside cities, the medical facilities in developing countries are often rudimentary. In addition, blood supplies may be inadequately screened. At the end of 2000, the number of adults and children estimated to be living with either HIV or AIDS worldwide was 36.1 million. Of these, 25.3 million are in sub-Saharan Africa, and 5.8 million are in South and South East Asia. It has been estimated also that about one-third of the blood supply in India comes from paid donors who are not adequately screened. It is therefore recommended that business travellers delay treatment until they can reach a facility where the safety of treatment can be assured. Many companies provide workers with their own supply of hypodermic needles and antibiotics and even some plasma substitute.

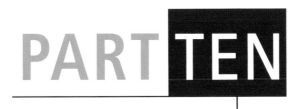

PART TEN

MISCELLANEOUS INDUSTRIAL
PROCESSES AND OTHER ACTIVITIES

28 Industrial processes

(a) Steel making

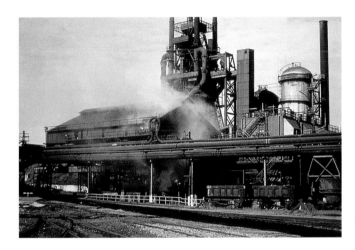

Figure 28.1 Ferro-manganese plant. Copyright Margaret Anne Harrison. Reproduced with permission.

What health surveillance should the workers in the ferro-manganese steel-making plant in the illustration receive? Manganese is a metal that is added to steel to toughen it. Absorption is via the gut (although it is not well absorbed) or by inhalation. Uptake is enhanced by iron-deficiency anaemia, and individual susceptibility is due to an interaction with iron metabolism. Manganese compounds are a mild irritant to the eyes, skin and mucous membranes. The inhalation of manganese by ore workers has been linked with a high incidence of pneumonia. The most serious consequence of manganese poisoning is the development of a form of Parkinson's disease. The final stage of the illness is characterized by akinesia and rigidity, muscle pains, paraesthesiae and speech impairment. Tremor is usually an intention tremor rather than a resting tremor. Biological monitoring is not generally helpful, so regular clinical assessments are required to detect early behavioural or physical changes.

(b) Car body repair

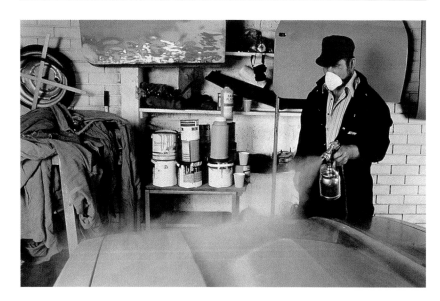

Figure 28.2 Car body repair: protection from exposure during paint spraying. Courtesy of the Health & Safety Executive, UK. Crown Copyright material is reproduced with the permission of the Controller of Her Majesty's Stationery Office.

There are many car body shops in the UK. Some are attached to large companies, but others are small concerns. The ingredients of car paint that produce the glossy finish are di-isocyanates, which are bifunctional molecules used to polymerize polyglycol and polyhydroxyl compounds to create polyurethanes. The paint is supplied in two parts, or 'two-packs'. The di-isocyanates are mixed with the polyols during the spraying process and the operative may be exposed to the di-isocyanates if adequate precautions are not taken. These chemicals are potent causes of asthma, bronchitis and, in some cases, extrinsic allergic alveolitis. Large companies usually ensure that spraying occurs in an enclosed, well-ventilated area and that workers wear air-fed full body suits. Unfortunately, some workers rely on inadequate respiratory protection and are employed in workplaces where health and safety regulations are ignored.

See also 'Occupational asthma' (page 77); 'Worker protection' (page 113).

(c) Foundry work

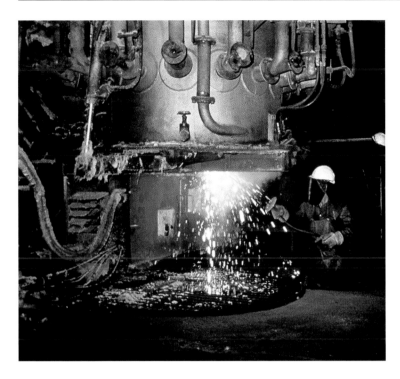

Figure 28.3 Foundry work: tapping a furnace. Copyright John Harrison. Reproduced with permission.

The man in the illustration is tapping a rock wool furnace. The process involves inserting a long curved metal pole into the bottom of the furnace to make the residue fall out of the bottom. The furnace is then re-charged. Rock wool is obtained from silicate-containing rock by heating it to liberate liquid silicates, blowing the liquid to produce fibres, and finally drawing out the fibres to the required length. Man-made vitreous fibres (MMVFs) are used as insulating materials as an alternative to asbestos. There are a number of structural similarities between MMVFs and asbestos fibres. MMVFs have been shown to cause mesotheliomas in animals. In most cases, the size of the MMVFs exceeds that considered to be respirable. However, pleural changes have been found in workers exposed to refractory ceramic fibres. To date, there is no evidence of an increased mortality from mesothelioma or bronchial carcinoma in workers producing MMVFs, apart from in the early production of rock wool. More data will be required to determine the safety, or otherwise, of refractory ceramic fibres.

(d) Quarrying

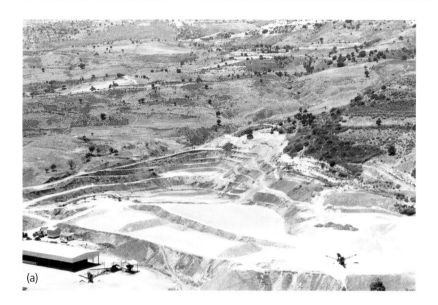

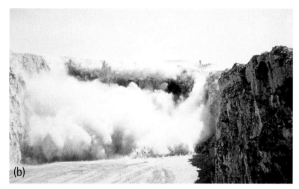

Figure 28.4 (a) and (b) Quarrying. (a) Copyright Nerys R. Williams. Reproduced with permission. (b) Copyright Margaret Anne Harrison. Reproduced with permission.

A number of prescribed diseases in the UK (diseases associated with specific activities in specific industries) are associated with quarrying activities. They include sensorineural hearing loss (Prescribed Disease Number A10), white finger (A11), carpal tunnel syndrome due to the use of hand-held vibrating tools (A12), pneumoconiosis (D1) and primary carcinoma of the lung in the presence of silicosis (D11). The quarrying and dressing of slate, sandstone and granite may lead to the generation of silica dust. There are three crystalline forms of silicon dioxide: quartz, cristobalite and tridymite. Pure quartz dust is a very potent cause of lung fibrosis. Slate contains a mixture of minerals, and the proportion of quartz varies from 35 per cent to 60 per cent.

See also 'Sound, noise and the ear' (page 25); 'Vibration (hand–arm and whole body)' (page 28); 'Silicosis' (page 90).

(e) Automotive assembly

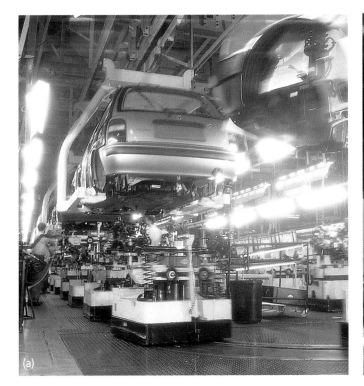

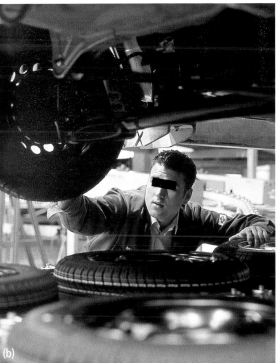

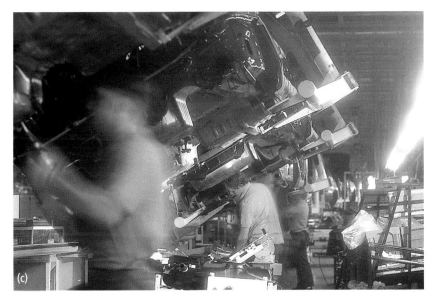

Figure 28.5 (a), (b) and (c) Automotive assembly. Copyright Nissan, Sunderland. Reproduced with permission.

Investment in new technology has led to the disappearance of many of the historical occupational hygiene problems. However, workers are still required to work on production lines, and work-related diseases may still occur. Production demands mean that they have to work quickly and repetitively, using the upper limbs and having to adopt awkward postures. A high level of physical fitness is required. Musculoskeletal problems may occur, which may be difficult to treat if the worker continues working. Modern industry is lean and efficient and there are no 'light jobs' for casualties – job modification or redeployment is usually not an option.

(f) Powder coating

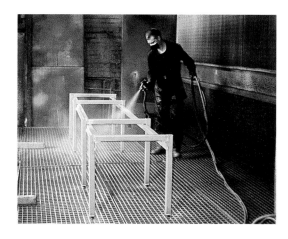

Figure 28.6 Powder coating. Copyright Nerys R. Williams. Reproduced with permission.

Metals and plastics can be protected by painting with a variety of materials – polyester, epoxy and epoxy polyester paints can all be sprayed onto a clean metal surface and provide protection against rust and the effects of weather. Some coatings containing tri-glycidyl-isocyanurate (TGIC) have been reported to cause outbreaks of dermatitis, with single case reports of occupational asthma also described.

(g) Shipbuilding

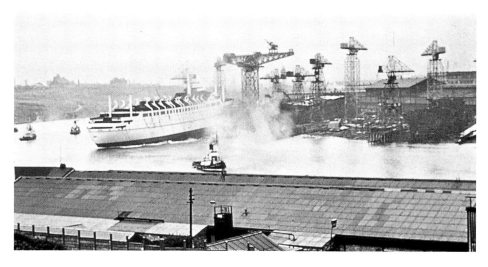

Figure 28.7 Shipbuilding. Copyright Print Services at the Robinson Library, University of Newcastle upon Tyne. Reproduced with permission.

Shipbuilding used to be a major industry in the UK. Building ships is associated with a large number of hazards and risks to health. The fabrication of metal structures and joining them together generated a lot of loud noise: metal often struck against metal, e.g. riveting. This also led to exposure to hand–arm vibration. Many ex-shipbuilders now suffer from noise-induced hearing loss and hand–arm vibration syndrome. Welding in confined spaces leading to the accumulation of toxic gases was also a problem. Welders had to have a high degree of physical fitness because of the conditions in which they had to work. Asbestos was used as an insulating material on ships.

See also 'Gases' (page 11); 'Sound, noise and the ear' (page 25); 'Vibration (hand–arm and whole body)' (page 28); 'Asbestosis' (page 82).

Chapter | *29* Other activities

(a) Food handling

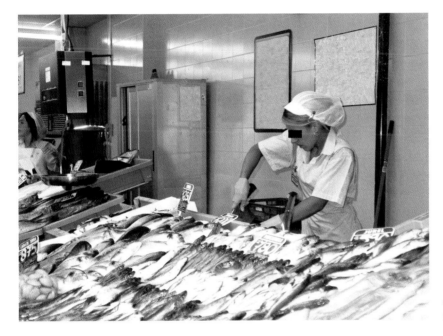

Figure 29.1 Supermarket worker handling fresh fish. Copyright Nerys R. Williams. Reproduced with permission.

Workers in the food industry have to adhere to stringent standards of hygiene to avoid contaminating the product. Diarrhoeal illness necessitates avoidance of food handling whilst symptoms continue and for 48 hours after their last symptoms. Ergonomic issues related to repetitive movements and manual handling are common, but the most frequent occupational problems in kitchens, canteens and catering establishments are slips, trips and falls.

(b) Occupational dysphonia

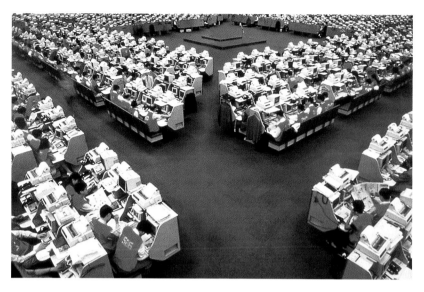

Figure 29.2 An early style of call centre. Copyright J.M. Harrington. Reproduced with permission.

Work in call centres has been postulated to lead to occupationally-acquired voice problems athough there is little evidence for the proposition. Call or contact centres that use email and methods of communication other than the telephone employ around two percent of the UK population although, due to costs, many centres are being relocated overseas. Inbound call centre workers may speak from predetermined scripts although it is usually the customer who has to provide most vocal input. Outbound (telesales) operators are more likely to use raised and excited voices and to speak quickly and for longer time periods. They, as a group, may be at a higher risk of developing voice problems than inbound operators.

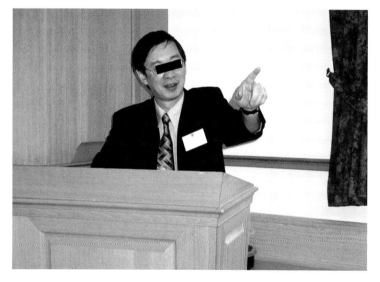

Figure 29.3 Occupational voice loss: lecturers and professional speakers are at risk of occupational dysphonia through repeated overuse of the voice. Copyright Nerys R. Williams. Reproduced with permission.

Individuals working in certain occupations, such as teachers, lawyers, the clergy, actors and singers, have been reported to have a high prevalence of occupational voice disorders ranging from minor changes in volume, quality and tone of the voice, through hoarseness, coughing and throat clearing to complete voice loss. This is thought to be due to overuse or abuse (i.e. screaming and shouting) and produces either temporary or permanent disability. Prevention is by ensuring workers reduce the amount of shouting at work, for example in teaching by appropriate classroom design and the arrangement of the more demanding or disruptive pupils near the front of the class. Other preventative measures include the use of microphones and sound systems, adequate hydration and avoidance of chemical irritants such as cigarette smoke.

Index